THE
OCD
FUNBOOK

Really?

Jimmy Huston

IMPORTANT! Rip this orderly and structured page out of the book. Tear it into little different-sized pieces. (Don't worry. This is *your* book.)

Throw the pieces away in lots of different places.

Doesn't that feel good? That's part of the fun!

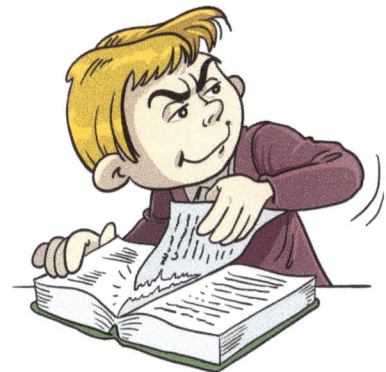

Cosworth Publishing
21545 Yucatan Avenue
Woodland Hills CA 91364
www.cosworthpublishing.com

For information regarding permission,
please send an email to *office@cosworthpublishing.com.*

Dedicated to Detective Adrian Monk

By the way, did you check to see what was on the other side of the page you threw away? It doesn't matter. It was just a dumb page out of a silly book. It wasn't important.

This page is totally unnecessary, too. Please tear it out and throw it away.

Don't be alarmed...

   ...but OCD can have harmful affects on people.

Don't be alarmed...

      ...but don't fail to act.

OCD can be serious.

      Don't be afraid to ask for help.

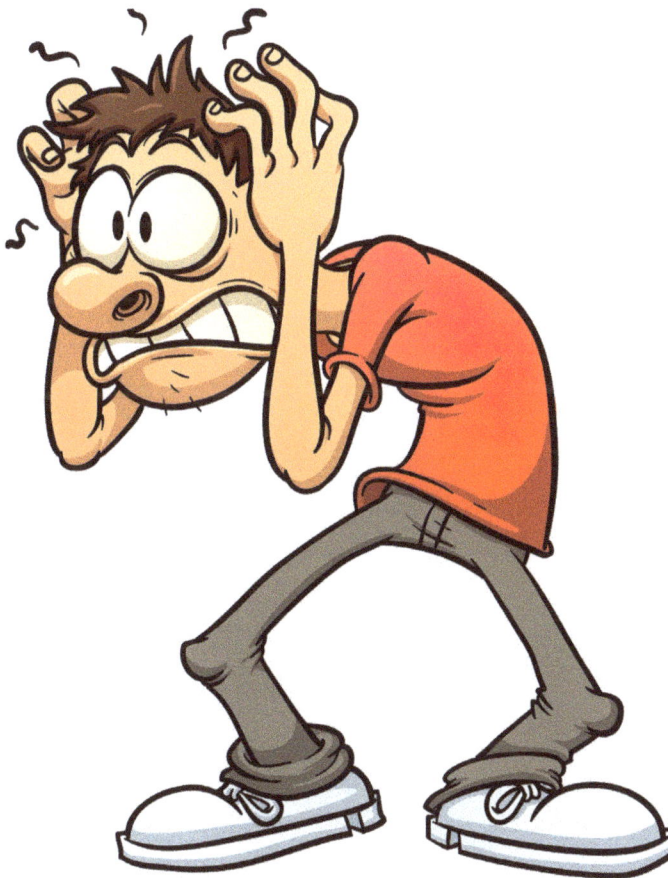

There is no need for a totally blank page. Tear it out. Throw it away.

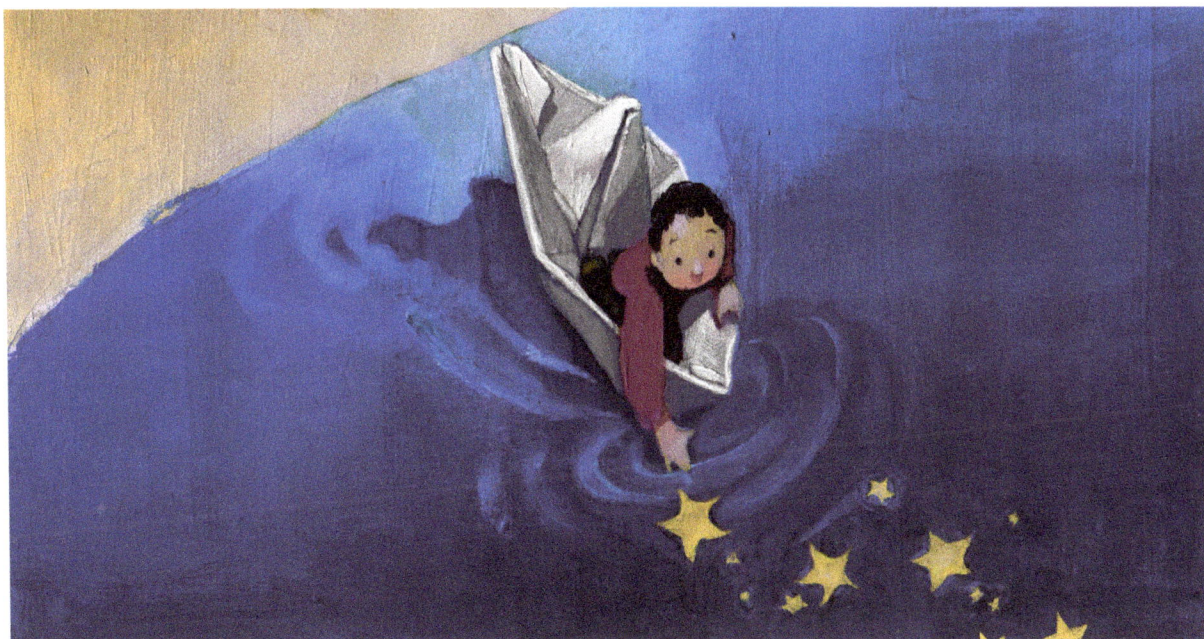

Introduction

Okay, this is serious. Don't tear this page out (yet).

OCD stands for Obsessive Compulsive Disorder.

It's right there in the name. Obsessive. Compulsive. Disorder. Three bad words.

For many people life with OCD is a strain, but there's a lighter side, too, and these behaviors can seem funny at times. People with OCD usually have insight into their issues and are aware of their quirks and foibles.

To be sure, OCD is not fun, but that doesn't mean that you can't have fun. That's what this book is for. You can laugh at OCD so you don't take everything too seriously. Life is good.

You can be happy.

Tear this page out, too.

Go ahead. Tear it out (after you read it).

Already read it? Then tear it out and rip it along the dotted line into four pieces.

Throw them away.

You may already think you have a problem. That's probably why you're reading this book. And, the people around you may either know or suspect something is going on with you. If someone gave you this book, that's a sign. You should pay attention, and maybe even thank them.

Let's start with the bad news. Sometimes these OCD thoughts and actions can lead to serious problems. That's why it's a good idea to learn about this before it gets worse.

Now the good news. There is help.

If you're having thoughts that create problems for you, thoughts that come at you over and over again, these may be what are called "obsessions." They aren't thoughts that you want to have, and they can be relentless. The types of thoughts can vary from one person to the next, but there are some that are common. Do you worry about germs and feel you need to wash your hands frequently? Do you worry that you've forgotten something important, like locking the door or turning off the stove?

Do you give in to those thoughts? If you obey those mental demands and act on them, those actions are called "compulsions." In a way, they are out of your control. They are not things that you would want to do — without the constant bombardment of obsessive thoughts.

So, it is logical to assume that if some of your thoughts make you need to do these unpleasant things, you should be able to conquer these bad thoughts with good thoughts. That's true, but it's harder than it sounds.

If it was that simple, this problem wouldn't exist. Everybody with OCD wishes they didn't have it. If trying to outthink OCD thoughts was enough, you could beat it yourself. But it's harder than that.

It's great to try. Fight OCD. Work at it.

But, the best thing you can do is get some professional help.

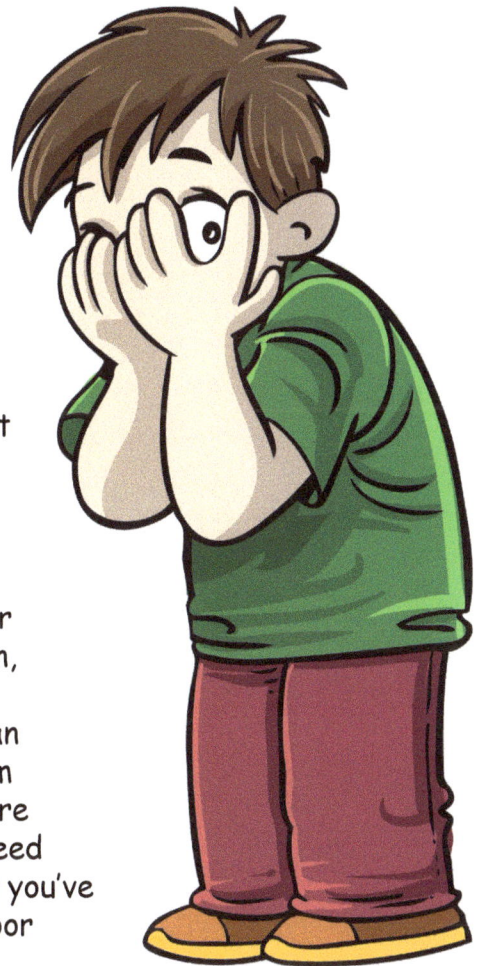

5

Now you can tear this page out. Get rid of it like you'd get rid of OCD, in a dozen pieces.

What is it?

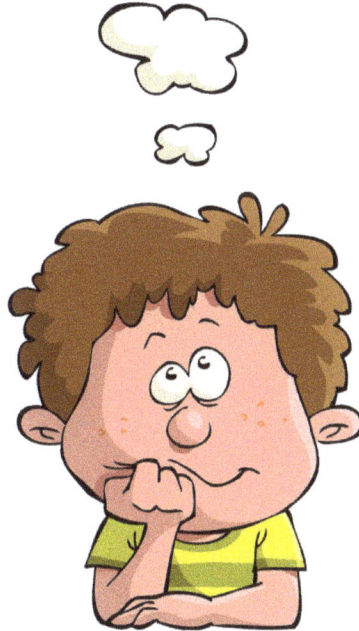

Obsessive Compulsive Disorder (sometimes called OCD) is just what it sounds like. People become obsessed with something that creates a desire for compulsive actions.

1. If you're thinking about the same thing over and over and can't stop, that's being OBSESSIVE. You may want to stop thinking about it, but you can't. The obsessive parts are the thoughts that keep barging in on you — thoughts that your hands are dirty or you are covered in germs. Perhaps you like to stack everything neatly. Maybe you have angry thoughts about people around you. An "obsession" might be as simple as counting something — over and over and over.

2. The COMPULSIVE part is the need to act on these obsessive thoughts. Maybe you wash your hands over and over. Maybe you start arguments or fights. Maybe you repeatedly check to see if the door is locked. Maybe you insist on having everything in an orderly manner, just the way you like it.

3. The DISORDER part just makes everything seem worse. DISORDER should be downgraded to DISTRACTION. If you have OCD, try to only think of it as Obsessive Compulsive Distraction. Don't you feel better already?

Now turn the page.

Did you turn the page? Are you sure? Did you go back and check? How many times?

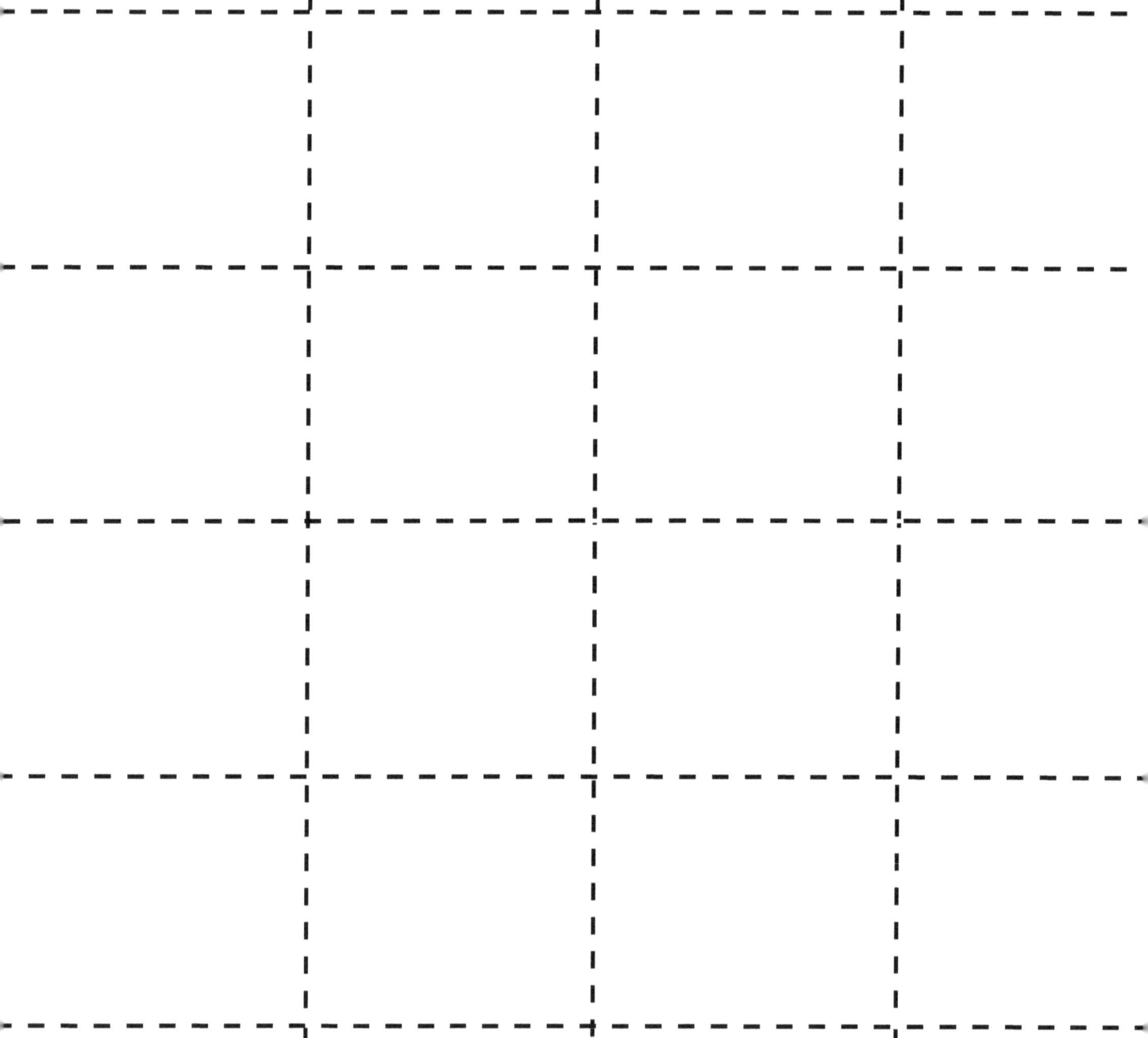

Maybe you should tear this page out, too, — before things get confusing. Tear it into 24 different pieces.   Then hide each one in a different place.

8

What is it?

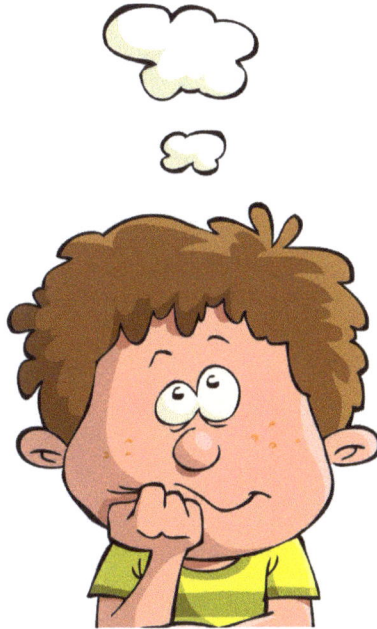

If you're thinking about the same thing over and over and can't stop, that's being obsessive. You may want to stop thinking about it, but you can't.

Sound familiar? Did you turn the page? Are you sure?

Okay. Enough of that. This is life with OCD, that we're now calling Obsessive Compulsive Distraction. It's very repetitive, very repetitive, very repetitive. And frustrating, frustrating, frustrating.

You'd like to skip ahead to the next page, or the next chapter, or the next book, but you can't. You're not exactly in control of yourself.

The obsessive parts are the thoughts that keep barging in on you — like insisting that things be in pairs, creating rituals for activities, or worrying about contamination or disease. It could be thoughts of guilt. Or panic.

Now turn the page.

This is an OCD test. If you have it, you know what to do.

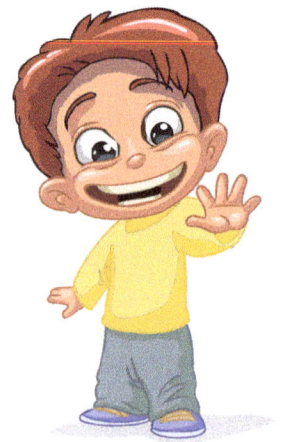

Yep. Tear it out. Throw it away.

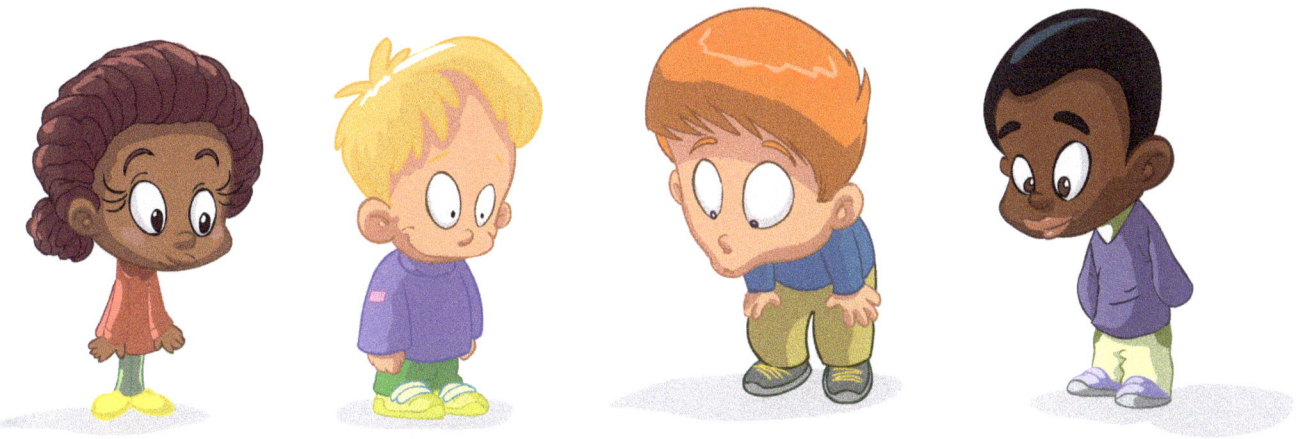

Who Gets OCD?

Anyone can have OCD symptoms, but that may not mean full blown OCD is present. You've probably seen people who occasionally do some seemingly OCD things, but not to a harmful degree. They just have OCD behaviors.

OCD can be chronic, and it can be genetic, so if your parents have OCD there is a slightly greater chance that you may inherit it. On the other hand, your parents may be a good example, showing you that you can live with OCD and have a good, normal life. (OCD is not contagious.)

About one percent of people experience OCD, and about half of those are considered severe.

Stress can make OCD worse. Sometimes trauma seems to trigger OCD.

You are not crazy or delusional. OCD is real.

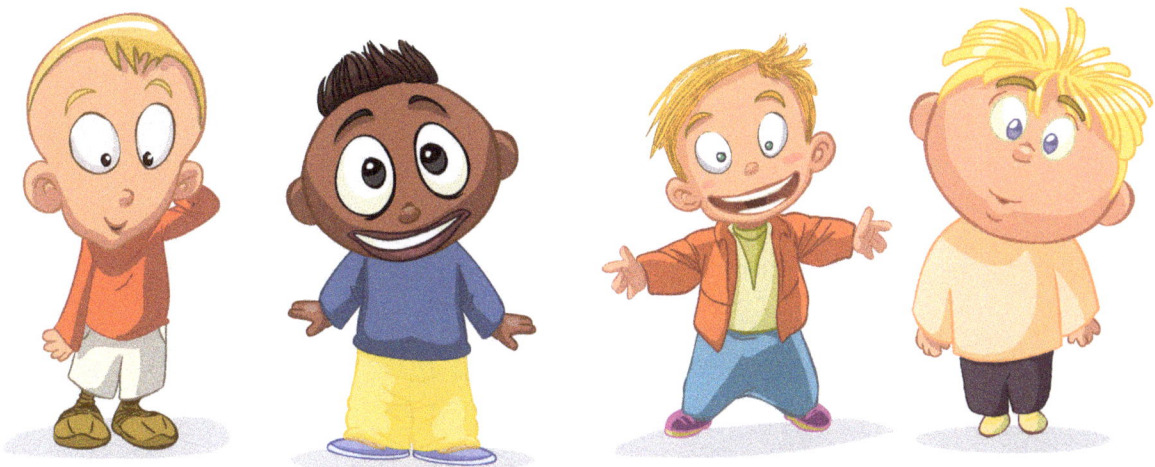

This page contains an invisible jigsaw puzzle. Tear it out, cut it into 27 different jigsaw puzzle pieces. Reassemble them into their proper places.

Throw away the entire puzzle.

Don't tear this page out. That would be obsessive. See? You're getting control already.

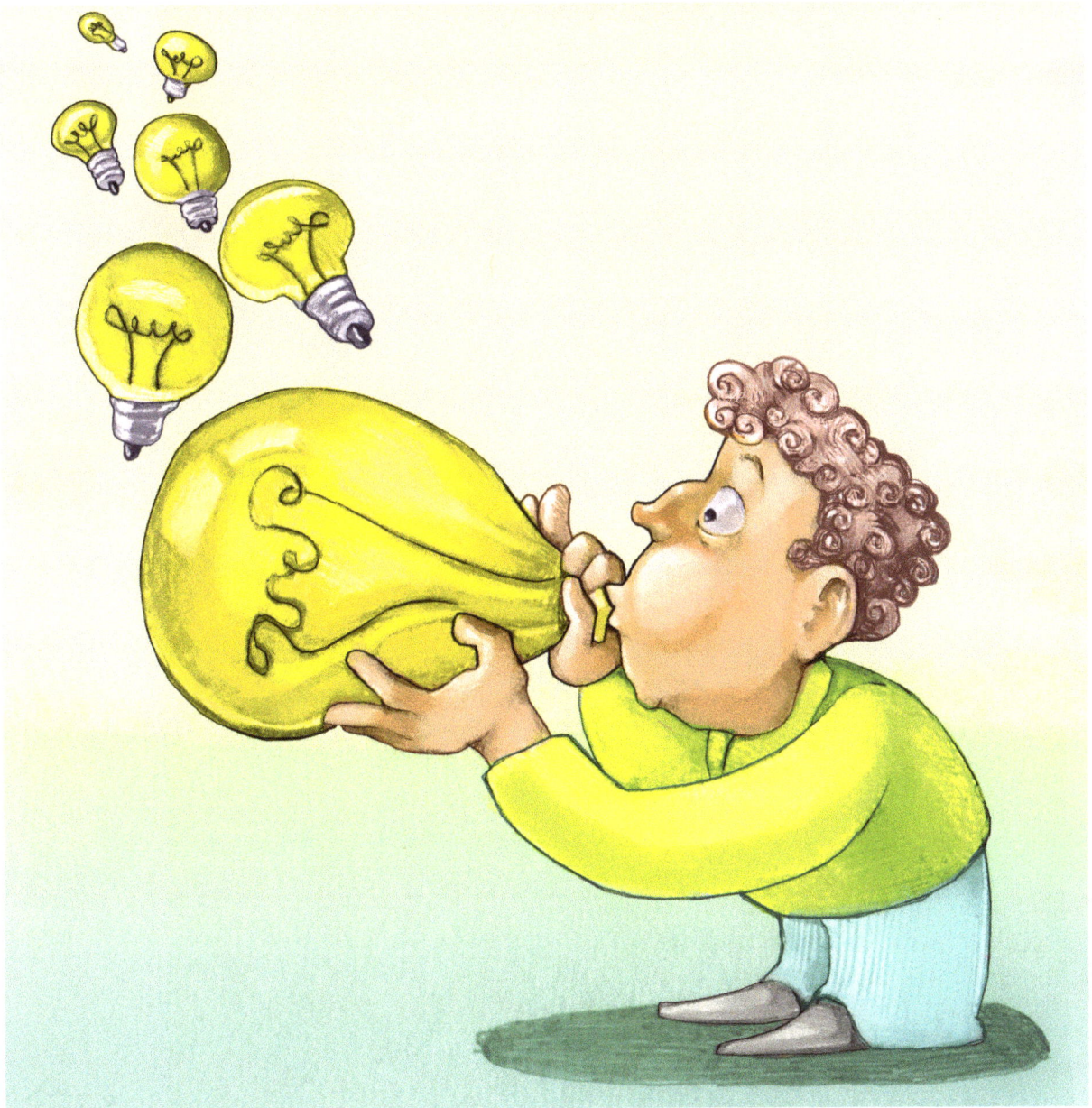

One way to think about OCD is to compare it to breathing.

We breathe constantly. Sometimes we control it, breathing in and out consciously. At other times we don't even think about it, and our brain takes over and controls it automatically.

Or, we can voluntarily stop it. Yes, we can stop breathing, completely and absolutely.

But not for long.

Okay, NOW you can throw this page away, too.

Did you tear it out of the book first? That's important.

It's not too bad at first.

Take a breath.

Hold it.

No problem.

For a while.

Hold it.

Hold it....

Hold it!

HOLD IT!

HOLD IT! HOLD IT! HOLD IT!!!!

HHHHOOOOOLLLLLLDDDDD ITTTTT!!!!!!!!!

But eventually...

WHHOOOOOOOOOOOOOOOOOOOOOOOOOOOOOOOOOOOSSSHHHHH!!!!!!

The air in your lungs comes bursting out, you suck in some fresh air, and you relax. Sort of...

You're not done. You're slightly out of breath, and you breathe a little more heavily than usual until you catch up. And, catching up doesn't mean you're done.

You still need to breathe. Your brain is always telling you, *"Breathe!"*

If you don't, the whole thing starts all over again. It never ends.

That's a little bit like OCD. It varies with individual behaviors but —

You can stop it. Absolutely. Whether it's a tic, or a grunt, or the need to step in a certain way, or to stack things in an orderly manner, or whatever...

Just stop it. No problem.

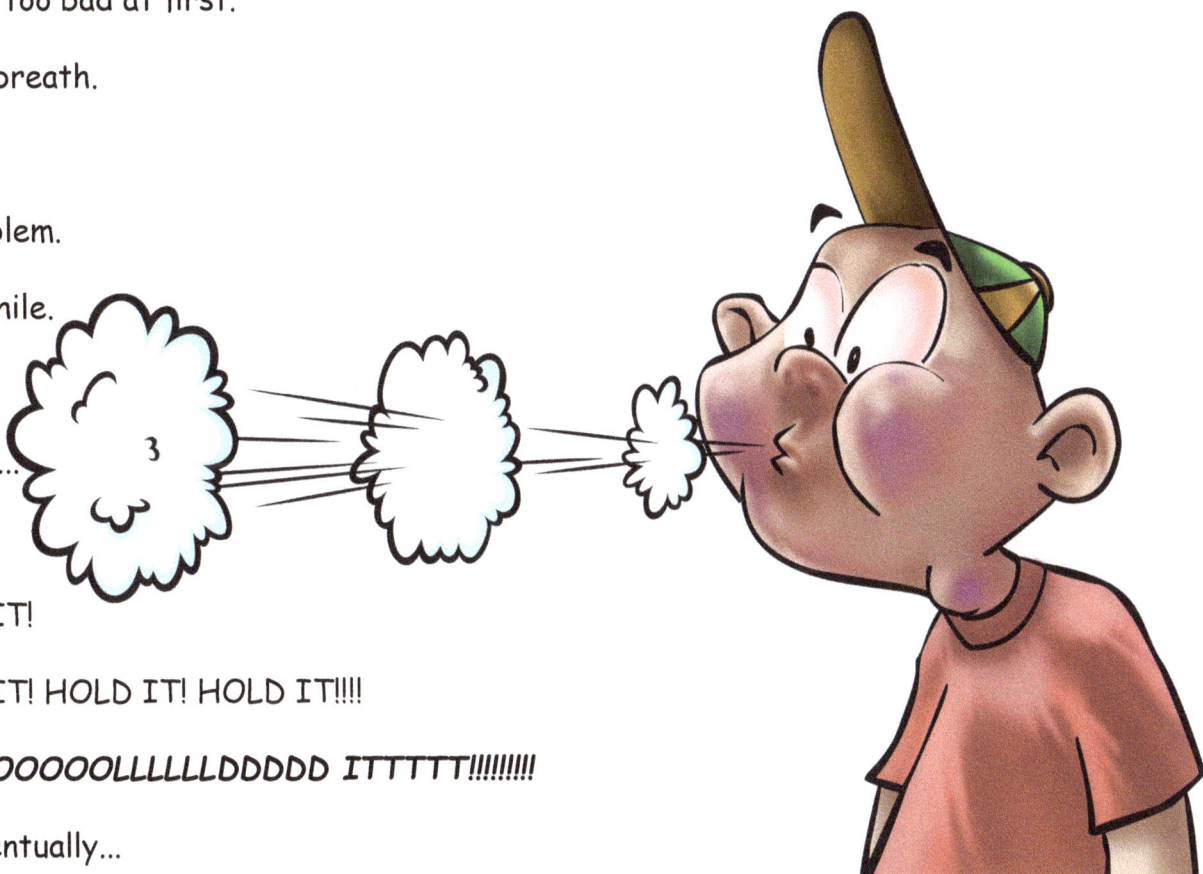

This blank page needs to be absolutely filled with little bubbles. Draw them. And smile.

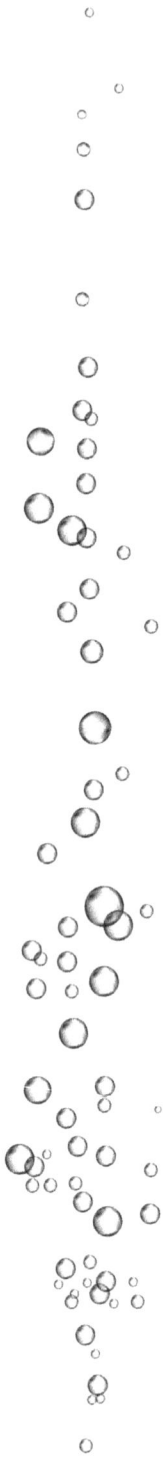

When you've finished, tear the page out. Rip it up into lots of little pieces.

At *first*.

But then, slowly, the pressure starts to build.

You can control it, of course.

It's no big deal.

You're smart. You're in control.

But it's still there.

It's in the back of your mind, but it's there.
It's definitely there.

The urge is growing.

The urge becomes a conscious thought.

Then it becomes a need.

That's what a compulsion is.

And, you have one. You have a compulsion.

Sometimes you can control it. For a minute, or a few minutes.

But sometimes you can't.

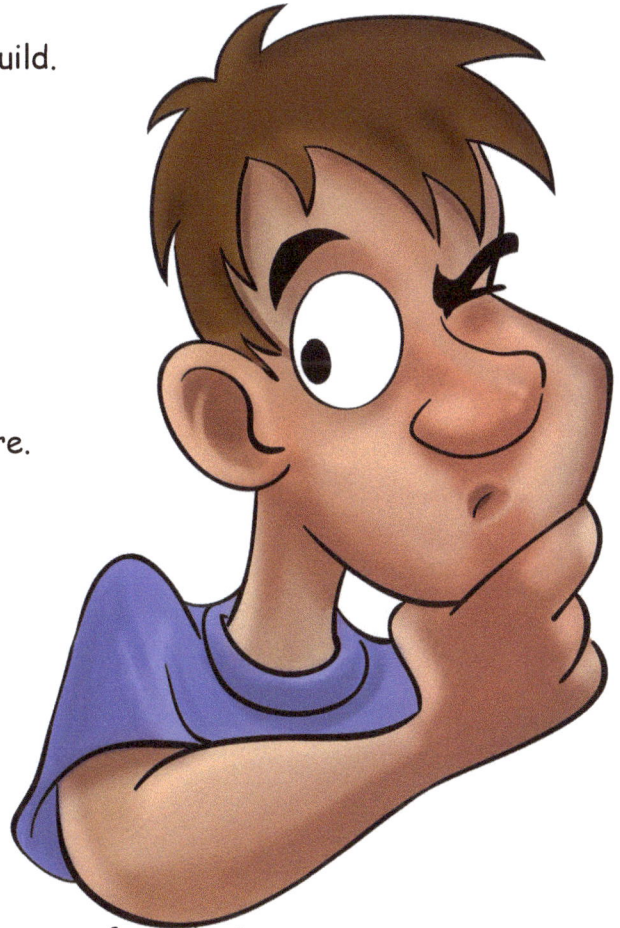

Maybe you're distracted and it takes over. It just comes out.

Or, maybe you give in, and you make a decision to let it happen.

Or, sometimes, you may not even be aware that you're doing it.

Like the breath in your lungs, the pressure grows and grows.
One way or another, it comes out.

It may seep out, or it may explode like a sneeze, but it's
definitely coming out.

And that's OCD.

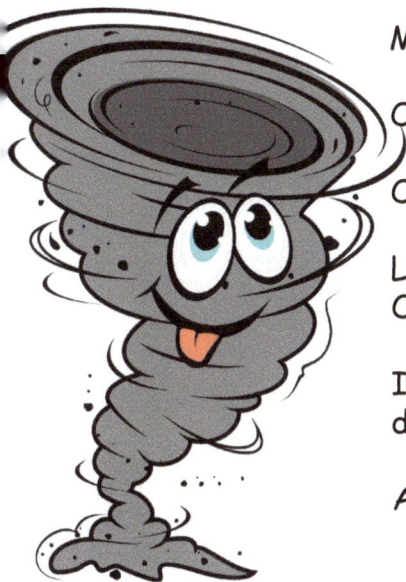

Fill this page with words. The content doesn't matter. The order doesn't matter. The size doesn't matter.

Carefully fill in all the enclosed spaces in all the letters. Rip it out, then throw it away.

Maybe a Better Example Is Blinking.

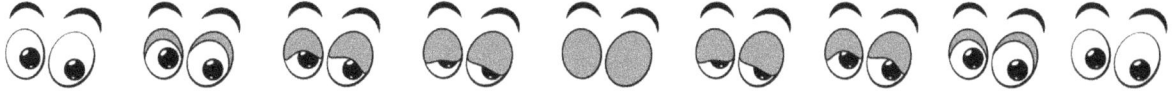

We blink all day long without thinking about it or even noticing that we're doing it.

Then, sometimes we think about it and we control the blinking.

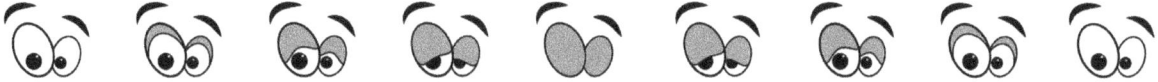

Or do we? The more we think about it, the more conscious we are of it, the more irregular it becomes. For some people — people with OCD — thinking about it takes over.

Should I blink? Should I blink now? Should I blink again? I don't want to blink. But I "need" to blink. And again. And again. Faster. Harder. Blink, blink, blink. Blink! Blink-blink. BLINK!

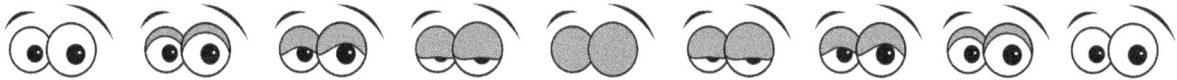

You're in control. But so is the blinking. Sometimes you win, sometimes you don't. You're probably thinking about blinking right now. Do you stop, or do you blink?

What about now? Blink? And now. Blink or no blink?

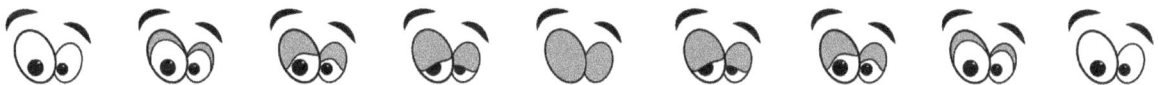

You have to blink sometime. What about now? Or later? How much later? Is it time yet?

Does your head jerk a little when you blink? Just a little bit?

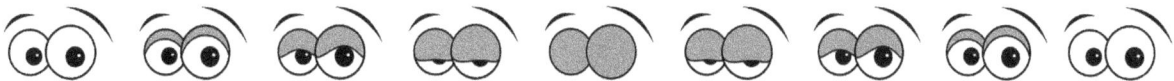

Well, it probably will now. Try it. Blink/jerk. Blink/jerk. Blink/jerk. Maybe you can just stop. Good for you. Some people can't. That's a compulsion. And people notice.

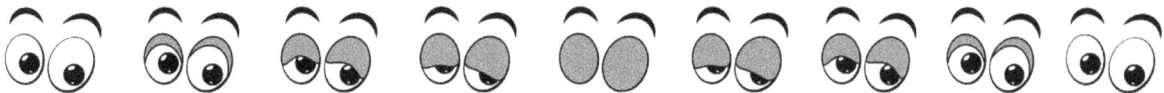

Maybe it's not even conscious. Maybe your OCD takes over and it just happens, without you really knowing it. Or if you notice, you don't care any more. It's just too compelling. That's OCD.

OCD Diagnostic Test

YES	NO	MAYBE	Do you have OCD?
YES	NO	MAYBE	Are you sure?
YES	NO	MAYBE	Do you have OCD?
YES	NO	MAYBE	Are you sure?
YES	NO	MAYBE	Do you have OCD?
YES	NO	MAYBE	Are you sure?
YES	NO	MAYBE	Did you just blink?
YES	NO	MAYBE	Do you have OCD?
YES	NO	MAYBE	Are you sure?
YES	NO	MAYBE	Was that you? Did you just grunt?
YES	NO	MAYBE	Do you have OCD?
YES	NO	MAYBE	Are you sure?
YES	NO	MAYBE	Did you clean your room today? Over and over?
YES	NO	MAYBE	Do you have OCD?
YES	NO	MAYBE	Are you sure?
YES	NO	MAYBE	Did you wash your hands?
YES	NO	MAYBE	Do you have OCD?
YES	NO	MAYBE	Are you sure?
YES	NO	MAYBE	Did you wash your hands *again*?
YES	NO	MAYBE	Do you have OCD?
YES	NO	MAYBE	Are you sure?
YES	NO	MAYBE	Are you still reading this?
YES	NO	MAYBE	Do you have OCD?
YES	NO	MAYBE	Are you sure?
YES	NO	MAYBE	Did you shower more than once today? More than twice?
YES	NO	MAYBE	Do you have OCD?
YES	NO	MAYBE	Are you sure?
YES	NO	MAYBE	Did you make a list today?
YES	NO	MAYBE	Do you have OCD?
YES	NO	MAYBE	Are you sure?
YES	NO	MAYBE	Are you getting angry or anxious?
YES	NO	MAYBE	Do you have OCD?
YES	NO	MAYBE	Are you sure?
YES	NO	MAYBE	Are people watching you?
YES	NO	MAYBE	Do you have OCD?
YES	NO	MAYBE	Are you sure?
YES	NO	MAYBE	Did you wash your hands *AGAIN*?
YES	YES	YES	Do you have OCD?

If you finished this, you are definitely OCD. Tear it into little pieces. Then get some help.

What are the symptoms?

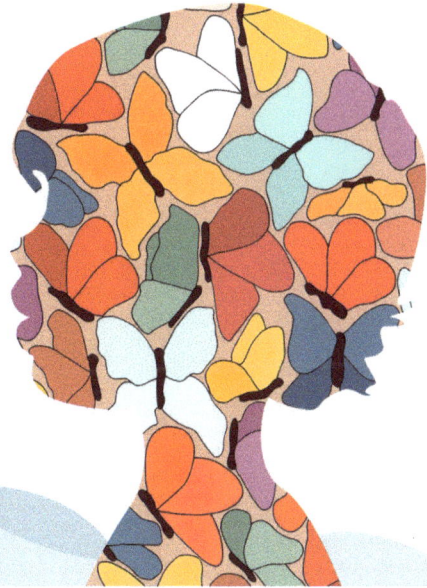

There seem to be a gazillion different symptoms that can occur with OCD. They don't complete a diagnosis, but here are some typical things to look for.

Obsessions are thoughts or urges, so they aren't apparent to an observer, but if you're having these kinds of thoughts it's worth noticing.

A big one is the fear of germs or things that might be contaminated. Some people fixate on having things in perfect or symmetrical order. Some people think about harming themselves or others. Maybe you create rituals around everyday activities. And, you feel an urgency about everything. Are you addicted to pain? Trouble sleeping? Hearing voices? Guilt? Panic? Sadness?

And doubt. Doubting that you locked the door or turned off the stove. Back in the 1800's OCD was called the Doubting Disease.

Behaviors are easier to spot, such as constant cleaning or handwashing. Or incessant counting, making lists, hoarding, and blinking. Alphabetizing things. Stacking things. Walking through doors repeatedly. Repeating things (perhaps under your breath). An obsession with numbers, including their taking on important meanings to you. Maybe you don't want to touch anything. Maybe you need to touch things repeatedly. Or both. OCD isn't logical.

Having one or more of these symptoms doesn't mean you have OCD. It could mean that you have a different condition that looks similar. Also, some people have OCD behaviors, but they don't actually have OCD. Having any of these symptoms isn't conclusive, so you should talk to a medical professional.

Wash this page.

You might want to tear it out first. Dry it carefully. Throw it away.

The odd thing about these compulsions is that they don't provide any real relief.

They nag, nag, nag at you, but if you give in and stack things or twitch or blink or wash your hands or check that the door is locked — it doesn't help you feel any better. You still feel like you need to do it again. So you stack things again or twitch again or blink again or wash your hands again or check that the door is locked again — and again, and again, and again. It's a never-ending cycle.

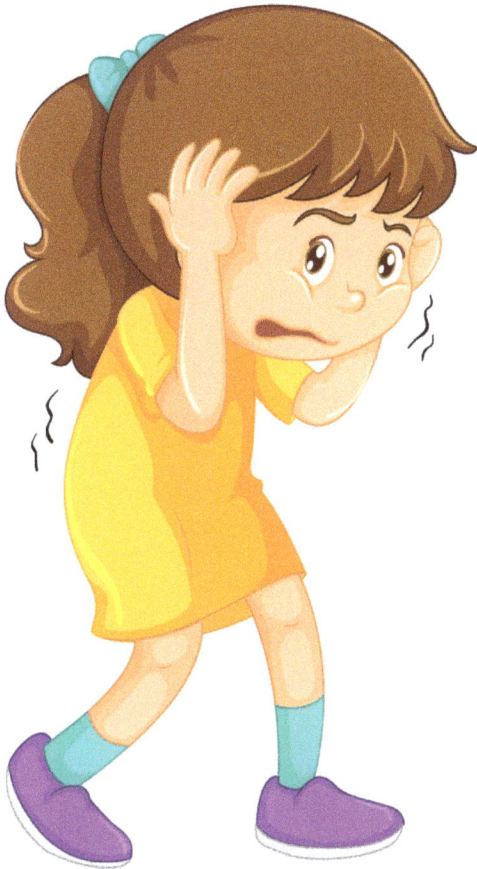

It's like when children walking on sidewalks amuse themselves by either never stepping on cracks (or they intentionally step on every crack).

Sometimes they rhyme along with something like, "Step on a crack, break your mother's back."

That would be a pretty severe penalty if it were true, but since the beginning of time, stepping on a crack has never actually broken any mother's back.

That's a little like the fear that promotes some OCD behaviors. It isn't real — or at least it isn't realistic. But it's there.

Can your fears come true? No.

You have to face your fears to learn they are unjustified and will go away without your compulsive actions.

Having OCD may be a little like having two minds inside of your brain. One pushes you to do something you don't really want to do. Maybe it's just a twitch, or a sound, or making something line up or stacking something. The other one doesn't want to do this. It may simply be a silent dialog, but it may be more than that, perhaps even a battle.

You're going to have to be an OCD warrior.

DO NOT READ THIS PAGE.

Really. Just skip the page without reading it.

There is absolutely nothing important here.

And there's nothing entertaining.

It's a complete waste of time.

It does show, however, (if you keep reading) that you are mired in structure and routine.

That's okay, but let's work on it. Just stop reading.

Now. Stop!

If you made it this far, there's still time to turn the page and keep your dignity.

Don't be a slave to reading one line after another.

Skip ahead.

Maybe even skip the next page altogether.

Really. Stop reading.

You've been warned.

There's nothing important here.

You're still wasting time doing something that's meaningless.

And that's sort of what OCD is like.

Well, you made it all the way. Too bad.

It means you're reading, but you're not getting the message.

Go back to the top of the page and start over — unless you've been on this one page for more than an hour.

In that case it's time to tear it out and move on.

Anxiety

Feeling anxious is at the heart of most OCD behaviors.

Worry, worry, worry. Your thoughts are spiraling.

You're trying to control a world that is out of control.

Everything is urgent.

It's constant overthinking.

Even the smallest things seem like an emergency.

It's common to have trouble sleeping.

Obsessive thoughts lead to unhappy feelings.

Nobody wants to have these thoughts.

They are cycles. They are distressing.

Untreated, OCD can lead to panic attacks, depression, anxiety, and shame.

It can ruin your life. Don't let it. Get some help.

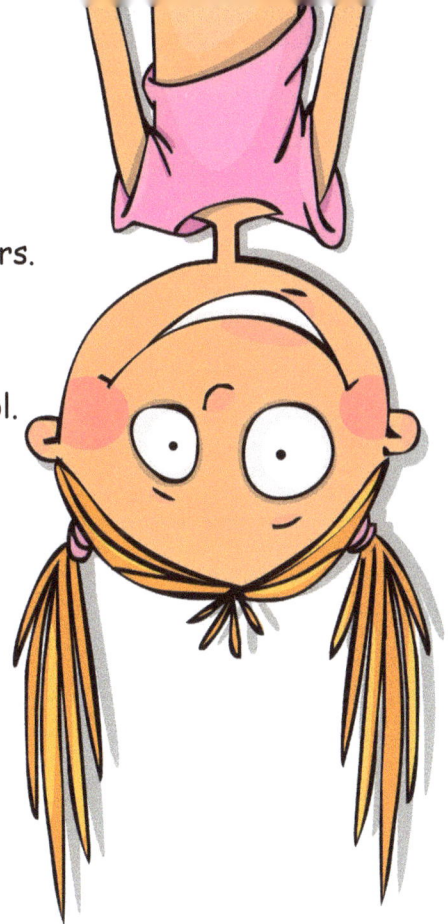

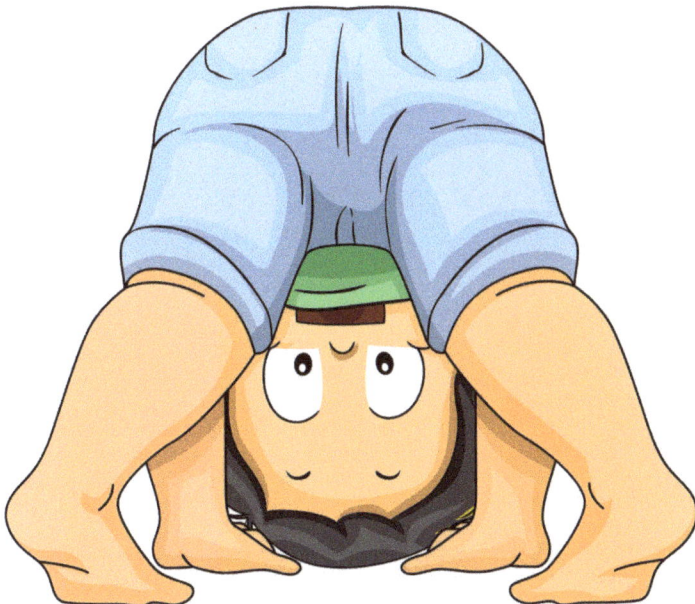

Write a note to a stranger on this page. Tear the page out and put it in a bottle.

Throw the bottle into the ocean. Or a river. Or a lake. Or a creek. Or a pond. But not a sewer or storm drain. And don't forget to put a cap on the bottle.

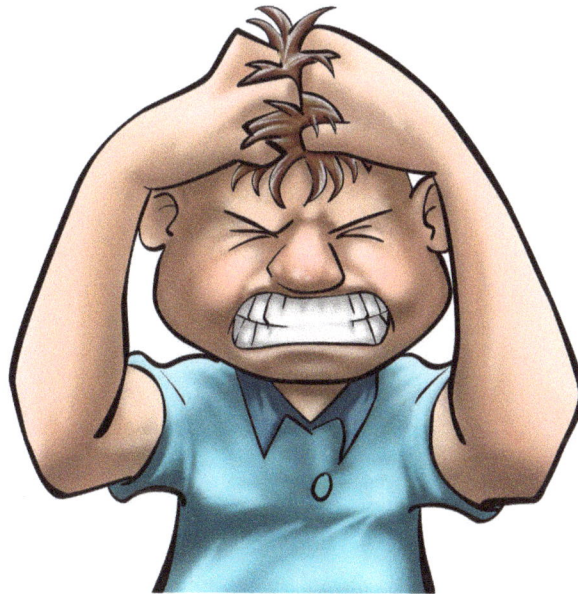

Thinking

OCD is marked by its own kind of thinking. It's thinking in circles. It's constant rumination about things that are both real and imaginary at the same time. It's worrying and worrying about things that shouldn't matter, but seem so very important. There's no relief.

All of the things that you're worrying about are coming from you yourself. They aren't based on true evidence. They're doubts. Did I do this? Is that going to happen? Should I have done something else?

They're coming from somewhere inside your speeding brain and they seem more real than the thoughts that you know to be true. Your brain is playing tricks on itself. And you're listening!

One of the things that sets people with OCD apart is that you know when you're doing OCD things. On some level you actually know what's true and what's doubtful. But — you just can't quite believe yourself.

When you lock the door or turn off the stove, tell yourself out loud. Or, if you have to, write a note to yourself. Put it in your pocket *with a time and date on it*. Take a photo with your phone as evidence. Find a way to believe yourself.

Ignore the OCD part of your brain. Trust yourself.

Trust yourself.

Draw a secret treasure map on this page.

Now bury a treasure somewhere completely different. Tear this page out and hide it where even you can't find it, just to be safe.

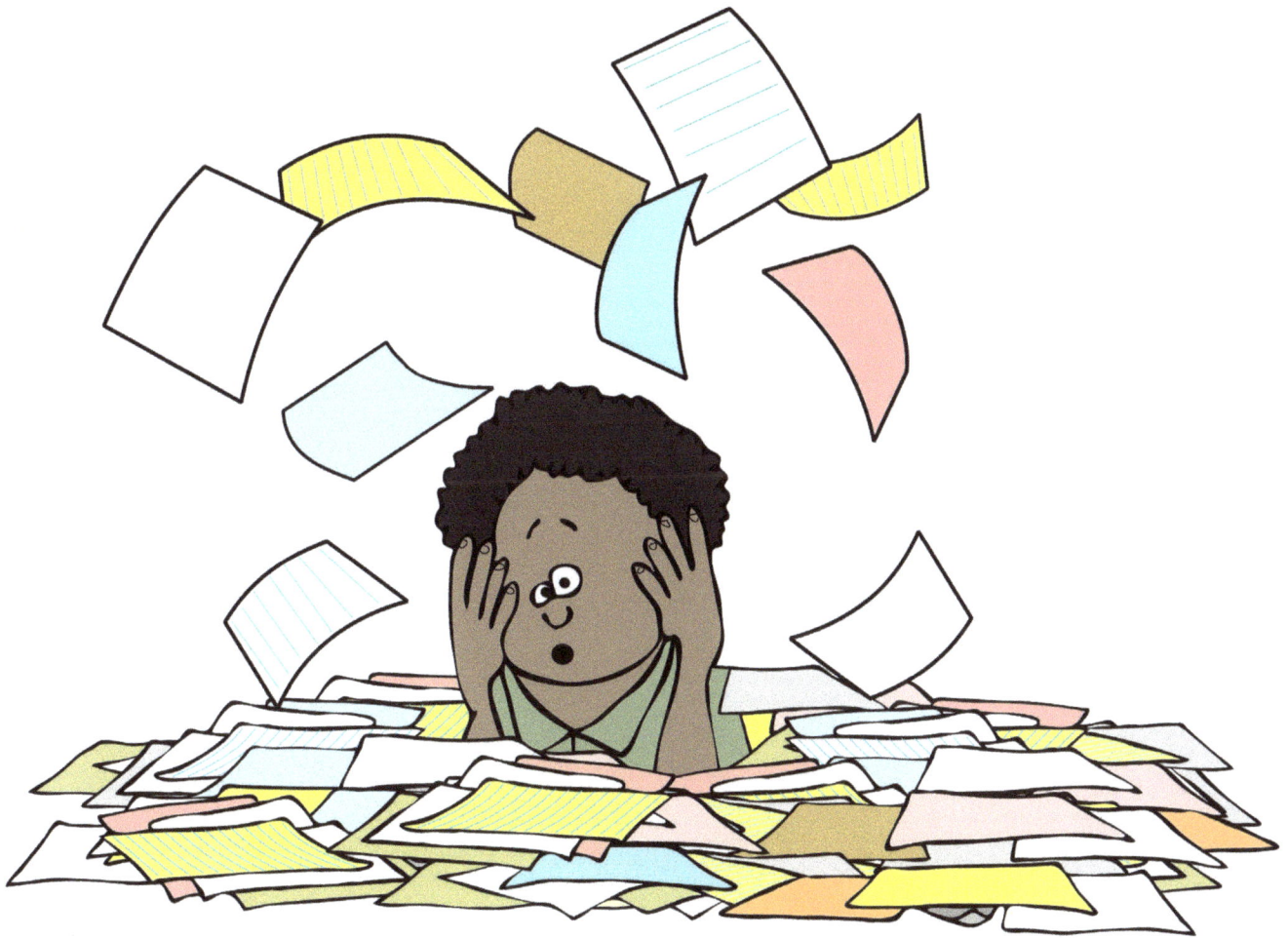

Orderliness and Symmetry

It's good to be neat. It's good to keep things orderly — whether it's clothes on hangers in your closet, or books arranged on shelves, or papers stacked or filed away. And it takes work to keep things tidy. But it can get to be too much.

If you fixate on a feeling that everything has to always be perfect, you're in for frequent disappointments and a lot of unnecessary work. When thoughts of neatness and orderliness take over, it can quickly become too much and overwhelm you.

Does everything in your life need to be even numbered? Or alphabetized?

Do you try to take the same number of steps with your left foot that you take with your right? Are you always counting things?

Those can be symptoms of OCD.

WRITE THE TOP TEN THINGS YOU LIKE ABOUT OCD

1.
2.
3.
4.
5.
6.
7.
8.
9.
10.
11.
12.
13.
14.
15.
16.
17.
18.
19.
20.
21.
22.
23.
24.
25.
26.
27.
28.
29.
30.
31.
32.
33.
34.
35.
36.
37.
38.
39.
40.   *Tear out this page and make ten copies. Fold them neatly and throw them away.*
41.
42.

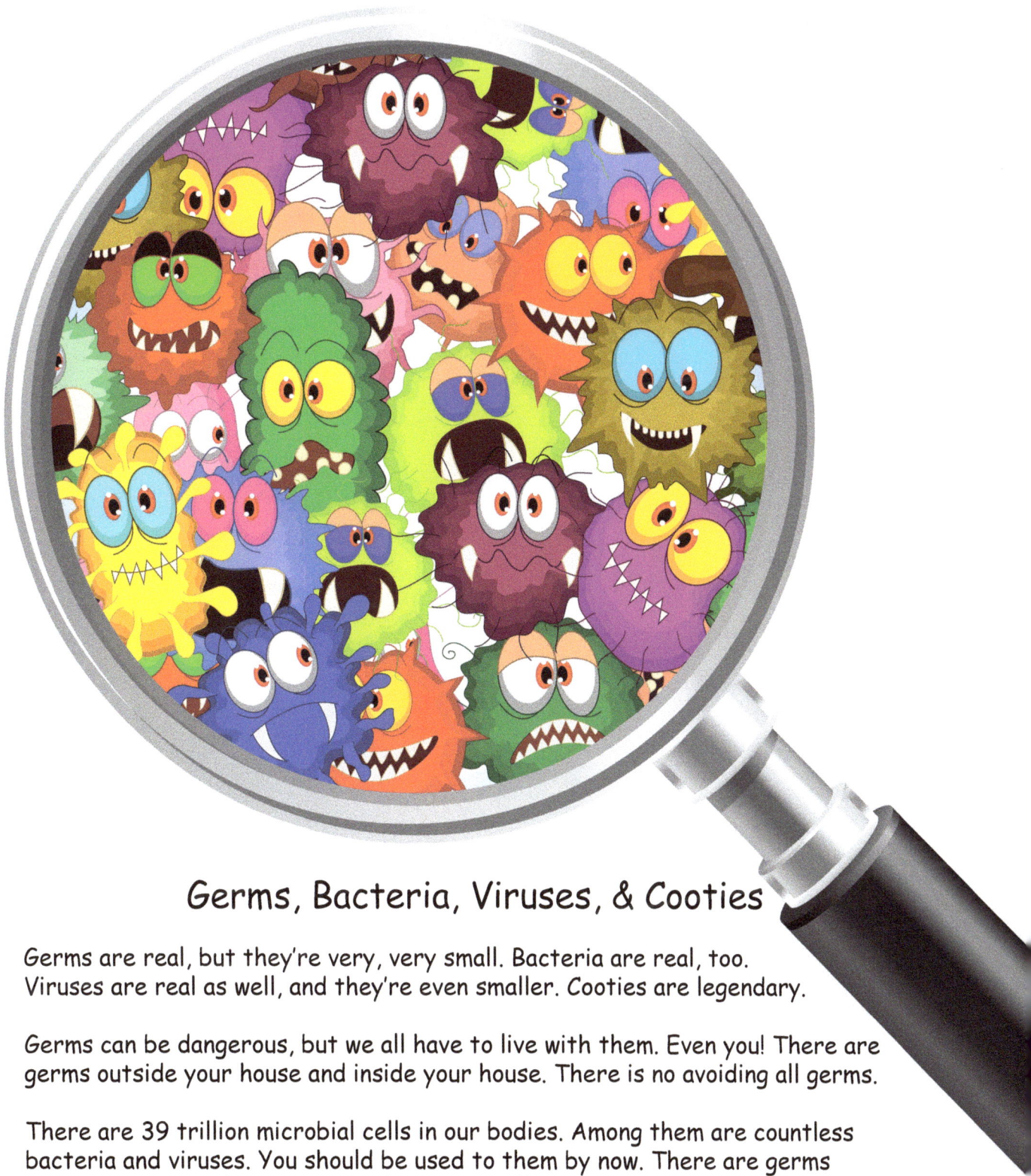

Germs, Bacteria, Viruses, & Cooties

Germs are real, but they're very, very small. Bacteria are real, too. Viruses are real as well, and they're even smaller. Cooties are legendary.

Germs can be dangerous, but we all have to live with them. Even you! There are germs outside your house and inside your house. There is no avoiding all germs.

There are 39 trillion microbial cells in our bodies. Among them are countless bacteria and viruses. You should be used to them by now. There are germs everywhere, or at least it seems like it, but all those germs aren't dangerous or the human race would've ended long ago. We're actually pretty strong.

Be clean. Be smart. But don't be ridiculous.

Rub your hands over these germs. Now, don't wash your hands.

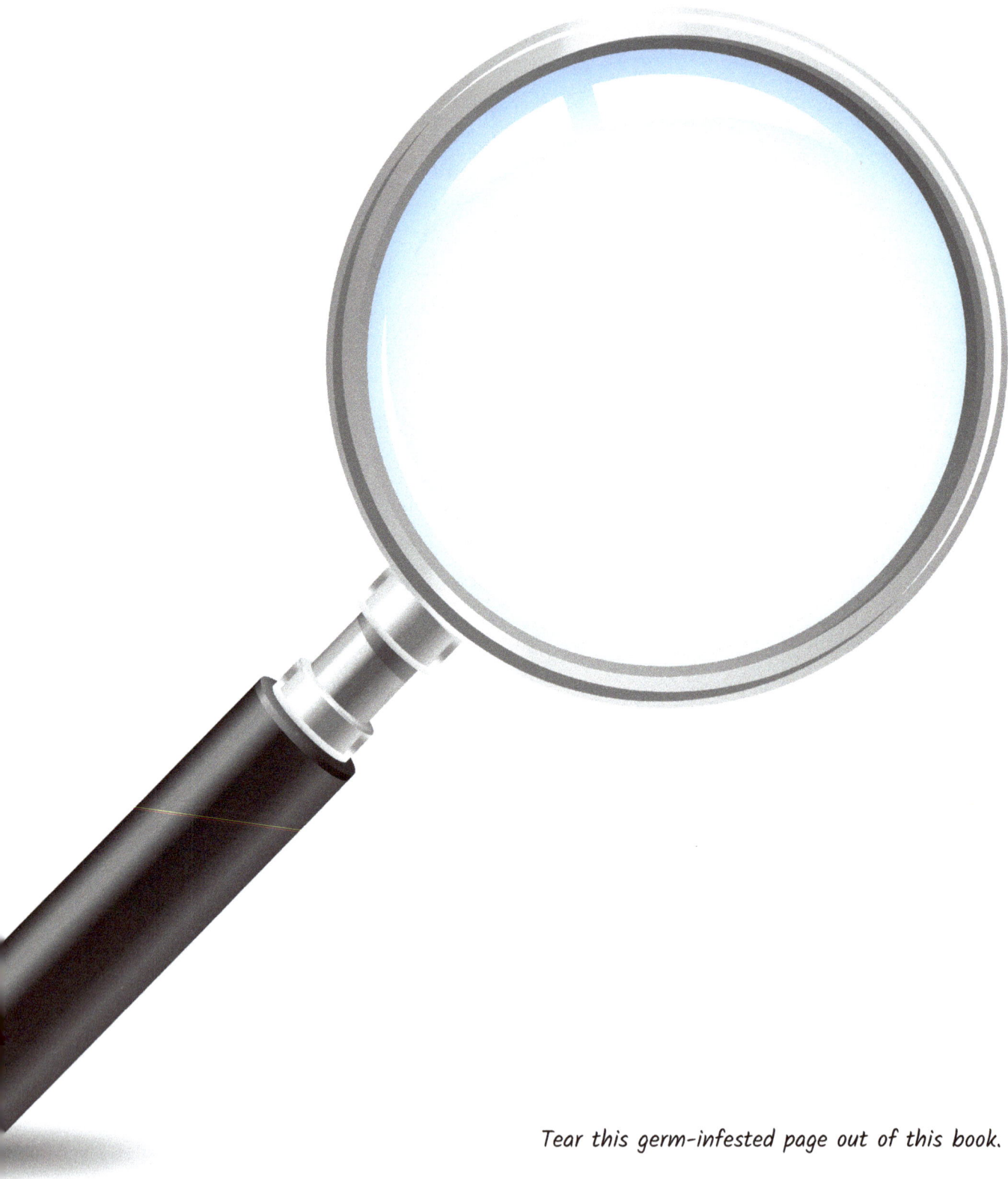

Tear this germ-infested page out of this book.

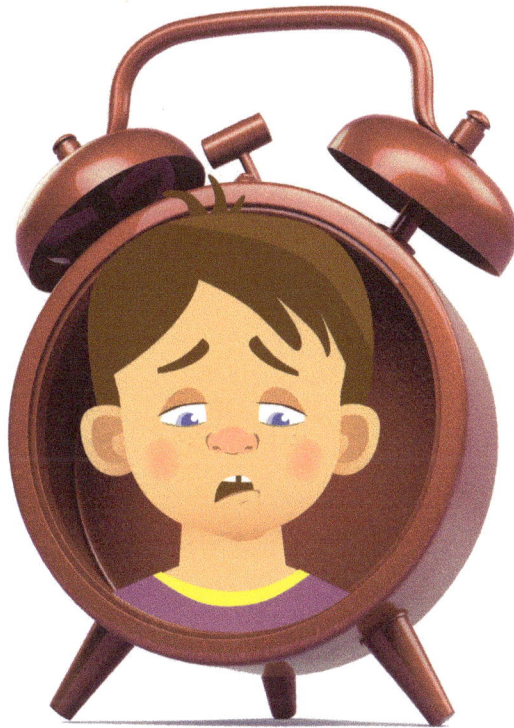

The Toc-less Tic

Many tics come with a toc. That's a different kind of tic. The OCD tic is a little movement (often jerky) that seems to come out of nowhere — usually in a series. It might be blinking, or it might be a twitch or a grunt.

These tics come out of the Tic Gland which is situated between your ears. Doctors often refer to this organ as your "brain."

Whenever there's one tic, there are usually more just behind it, trying to get out.

You can feel it coming. You're getting along perfectly fine when you notice a hint of a tic trying to get out. You try to ignore it, but you can't. It just gets more and more bothersome, insisting that you act out the tic.

It's a little like going to the bathroom. Initially, everything is fine and normal. No need to go to the bathroom at all. Then, eventually, you get that nagging feeling that something is coming. You don't have to do anything about it. You can even ignore it — for the moment — but eventually that feeling changes. It gets a little more noticeable, maybe a bit insistent, but it's still under control. But — already you know — you're definitely going to have to go to the bathroom. And, like it or not, you are definitely going to go to the bathroom pretty soon.

But you can't flush away tics. You're going to need to get help.

QwErTyUiOpAsfGhJkLzXcVbNmqWeRtYuIoPaSdFgHjKlZxcVbnM
qwertyuioopasdfghjklzxcvbnmQWERTYUIOASDFGHJKLZXCVBNM
QWERTYUIPASDFGHJKLZXCVBNMqwertyuioopasdfghjklzxcvbnm
QwErTyUiOpAsDfGhJkLzXcVbNmqWeRtYuIoPaSdFgHjlZxcVbnM
wertyuioopasdfghjklzxcvbnmQWERTYUIOPASDFGHJKLZXCVBNM
QWERTYUIOPASDFGHJKLZXCVBNMqwertyuiopasdfghjklzxcvbnm
QwErTyUiOpAsDfGhJkLzXcVbNmqWeRtYuIoPaSdFgHjKlZxcVbn
qwertyuioopasdfghjklzxcvbnmQWERTYUOPASDFGHJKLZXCVBNM
QWERTYUOPASDFGHJKLZXCVBNMqwertyuioopasdfghjklzxcvbnm
QwErTUiOpAsDfGhJkLzXcVbNmqWeRtYuIoPaSdFgHjKlZxcVbnM
qwertyuioopasdfghjklzxcbnmQWERTYUIOPASDFGHJKLZXCVBNM
QWERTYUIOPASDFGHJKLZXCVBNMqwertyuiooasdfghjklzxcvbnm
QwErTyUiOpAsDfGhJkLzXcVbNmqeRtYuIoPaSdFgHjKlZxcVbnM
qwertyuioopasdfghjklzxcvbnmQWETYUIOPASDFGHJKLZXCVBNM
QWRTYUIOPASDFGHJKLZXCVBNMqwertyuioopasdfghjklzxcvbnm
QwErTyUiOpAsDfGhJkLzXcVbNmqWeRtYuIoPaSdFgHjKlxcVbnM
qwertyuioopasdfghjklzxcvbnmQWERTYUIOPASDFHJKLZXCVBNM
QWERTYUIOPASDGHJKLZXCVBNMqwertyuioopasdfghjklzxcvbnm
QwErTyUiOAsDfGhJkLzXcVbNmqWeRtYuIoPaSdFgHjKlZxcVbnM
qwertyuioopasdfghjkzxcvbnmQWERTYUIOPASDFGHJKLZXCVBNM
QWERTYUIOPASDFGHKLZXCVBNMqwertyuioopasdfghjklzxcvbnm
QwErTyUiOpAsDfGhJkLzXcVbNmqWeRtYuIoaSdFgHjKlZxcVbnM
qwertyuioopasdfghjklzxcvbnmQWERTYUIOPASDFGHJKLZCVBNM
QWERTYUIOPASDFGHJKLZXCVBNMqwertyuiooopasdfgjklzxcvbnm
QwErTyUiOpAsDfGhJkLzXcVbNmqWeRtYuIoPaSdFgHjKlZxcVBM
qwertyuiooopsdfghjklzxcvbnmQWERTYUIOPASDFGHJKLZXCVBNM
QWERTYUIOPSDFGHJKLZXCVBNMqwertyuiooopasdfghjklzxcvbnm
QwErTyUiOpAsDfGhJkLzXcVbNmWeRtYuIoPaSdFgHjKlZxcVbnM
qwertyuiooopasdfghjklxcvbnmQWERTYUIOPASDFGHJKLZXCVBNM

Make a list of the missing letters. Rip the page out and destroy it. And the list, too.

Hoarding

Do you keep taking the little packets of ketchup or sugar from restaurants? Do you have lots of matchbooks from everywhere you've been?

Is your closet full? Things under the bed? Drawers stuffed? Boxes everywhere, filled with you don't remember what? It's not collecting. It's not saving. Those aren't mementos. You're hoarding.

If you keep lots and lots of things that you don't need — things that are obsolete or broken or worthless — you're hoarding. It's not harmful, but it puts your energy into the wrong things. It's an OCD sign.

Touch each spot at least once, touching as many as you can at one time.

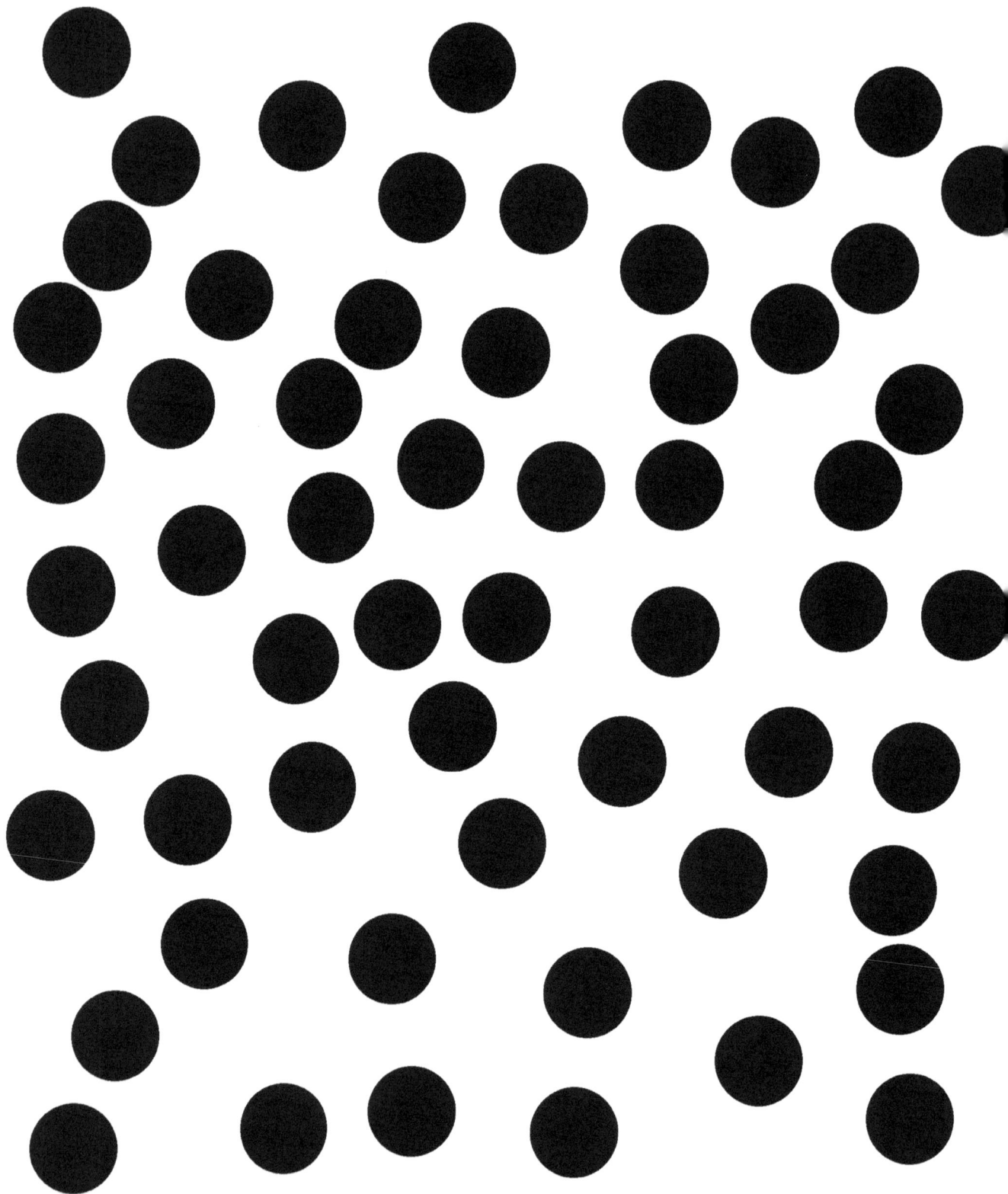

Ewwww. This page has been touched all over. Tear it out, wash it, and throw it away.

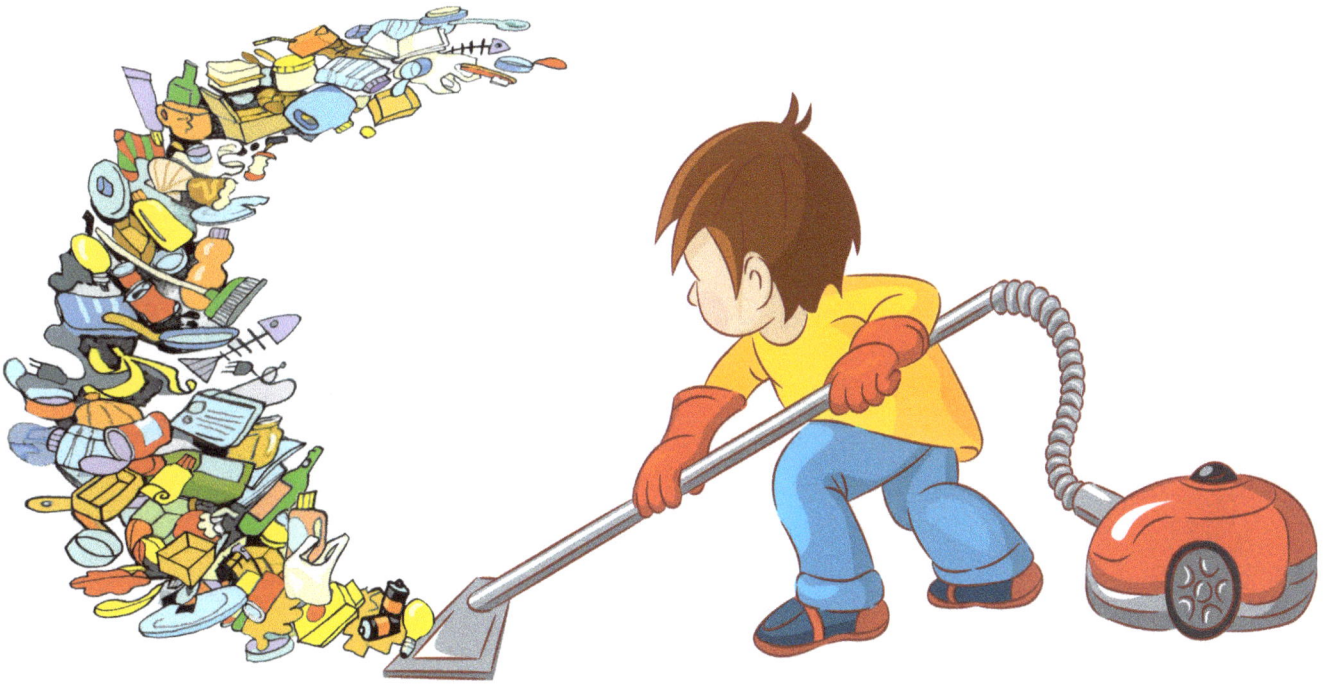

Cleaning, Cleaning, & More Cleaning

You've been told to keep your room clean. So now you're doing it, and you're doing a great job. What's the problem?

Keeping things clean is great. But, if you're going overboard — if you're spending too much time worrying about keeping it clean — if you insist that things always need to be perfect (and you think about it a lot) that may be obsessive.

If you're always worried about "contamination" and are constantly washing things — and it's taking the place of other things in your life — that may be compulsive.

Does clutter cause you stress? Do you need to stack things or put them in rows? Do you alphabetize things or align them in pairs? Do you wash things (including yourself) repeatedly?

Most people like having things clean and neat. Maybe clothes should be folded neatly or hung in a closet. Perhaps things are best stacked in cabinets or on shelves. If your desk is organized, that's usually good. Are your toys put away in an orderly manner? Good for you. But don't go nuts over it.

When compulsions always want more and more cleanliness, more order, more stacking — when cleanliness demands start to take over, that can be a sign of OCD. Just relax. Every now and then, enjoy the dirt.

Getting frustrated? Take out all your anger on this stupid page.

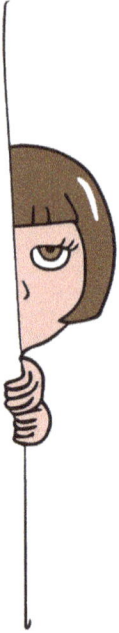

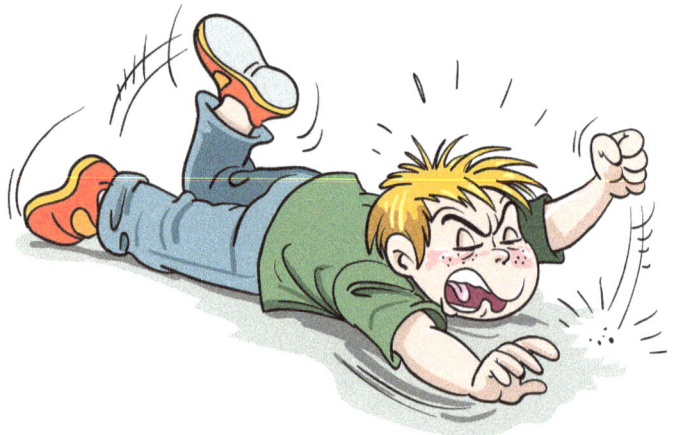

Rip the page out and tear it into small OCD pieces. Stack them neatly in the trash.

And Other Things OCD

Some people have an obsession with things like...

...aggressive thoughts.

...an addiction to pain.

...bathroom anxieties.

...contamination fears.

...fear of leaving the house.

...fear of crowds.

...hypochondriac tendencies — meaning they believe they have a physical illness when they do not.

...a general unhappiness with body image and appearance (body dysmorphic disorder). You don't like the way you look. Or, you HATE the way you look.

...fixating on the body's physical odor.

...skin picking.

...hair pulling, twisting, and eating.

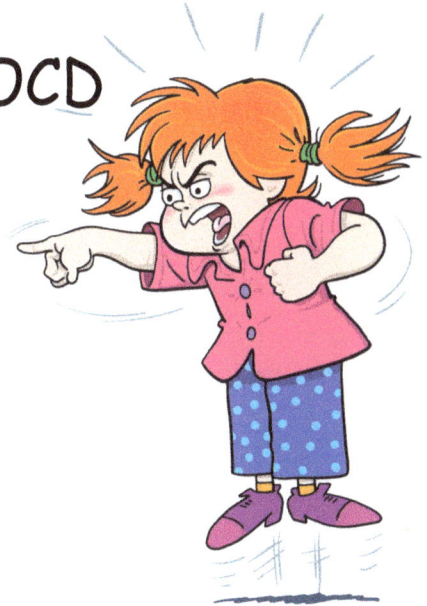

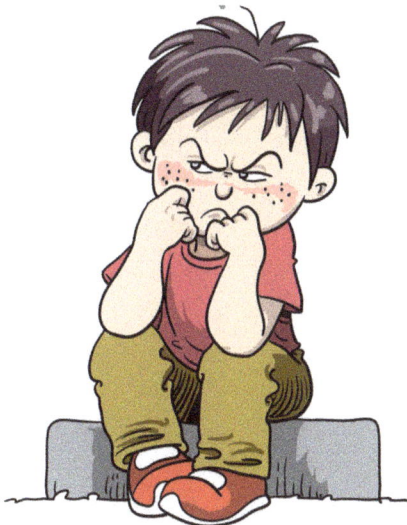

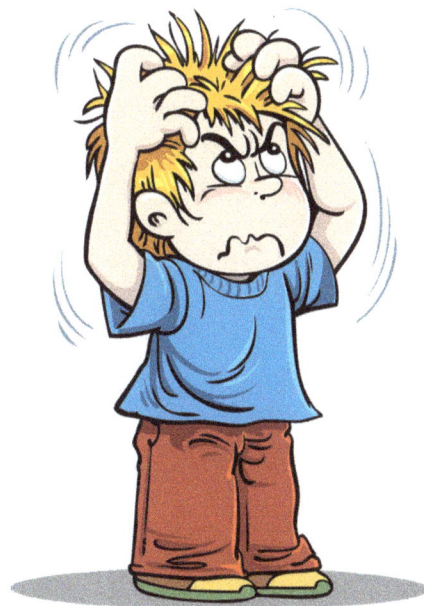

Doctors believe that OCD is caused by an inflammation of the part of the brain called the amygdala. Its normal job is interpreting threats. Make a list of everything that you believe threatens you.

1. _____
2. _____
3. _____
4. _____
5. _____
6. _____
7. _____
8. _____
9. _____
10. _____
11. _____
12. _____
13. _____
14. _____
15. _____
16. _____
17. _____
18. _____
19. _____
20. _____
21. _____
22. _____
23. _____
24. _____
25. _____
26. _____
27. _____
28. _____
29. _____
30. _____
31. _____
32. _____
33. _____
34. _____
35. _____

Get rid of your threats. Tear this page out and bury it somewhere deep.

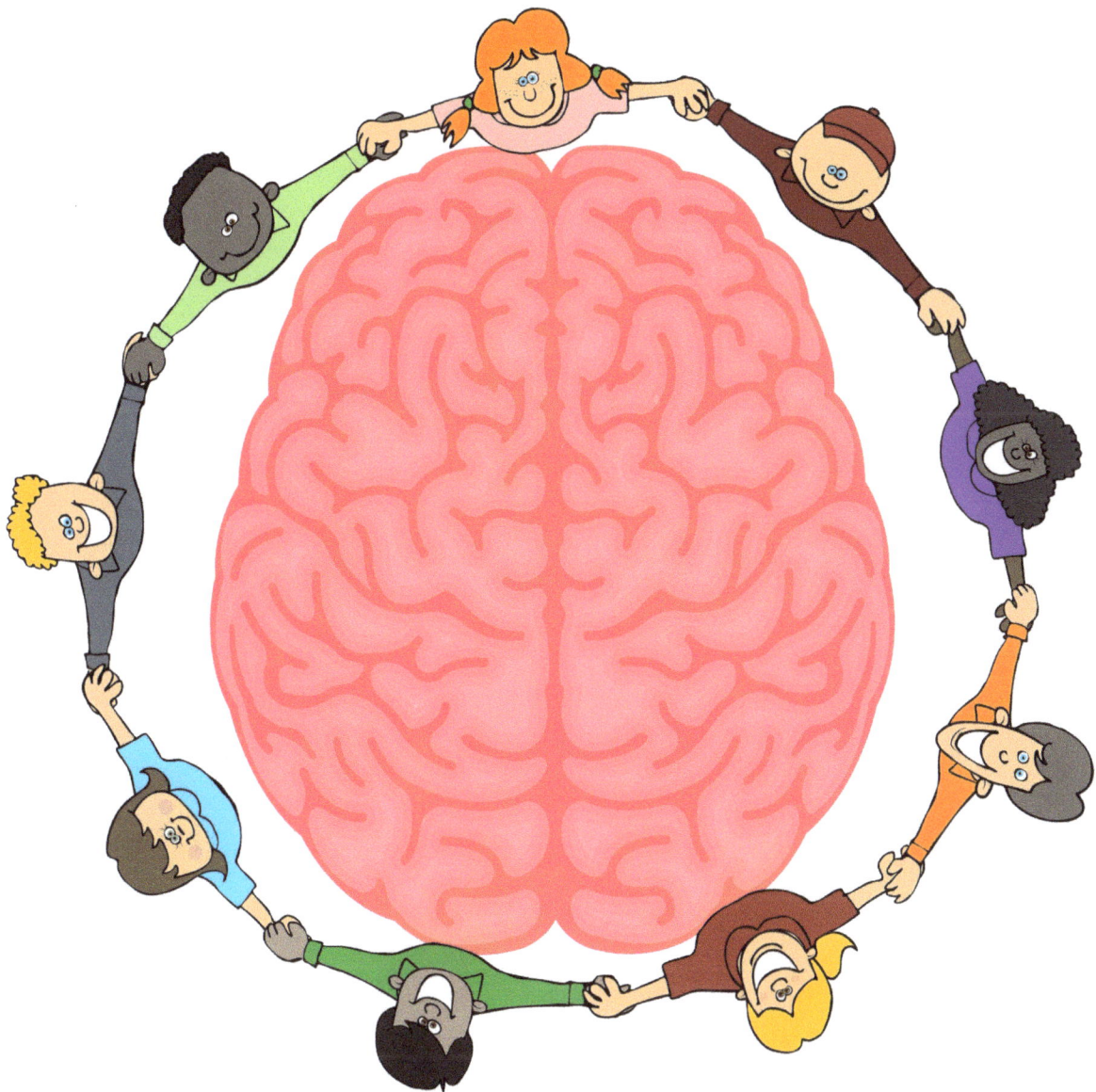

Everybody knows that the brain is the center of everything in a person — good or bad — physical or mental. Certainly when discussing OCD, the brain usually comes up. But there is no OCD gland in the brain. You can't see the OCD part in an X-ray or MRI. But we know it's there.

That's because — even with all the science — the brain doesn't really explain everything. Your actual brain is just a bunch of unremarkable spongy stuff, but the important parts are electrical or chemical. Nobody can see them, and we don't *really* understand them, which sort of means that they're almost mystical, but they're definitely there.

Sure the brain controls some things in the body that are understandable, but a lot of it is mysterious.

How many words can you cram onto this page? Write them, then count them.

Tear each word into a separate piece of paper and then alphabetize them all.

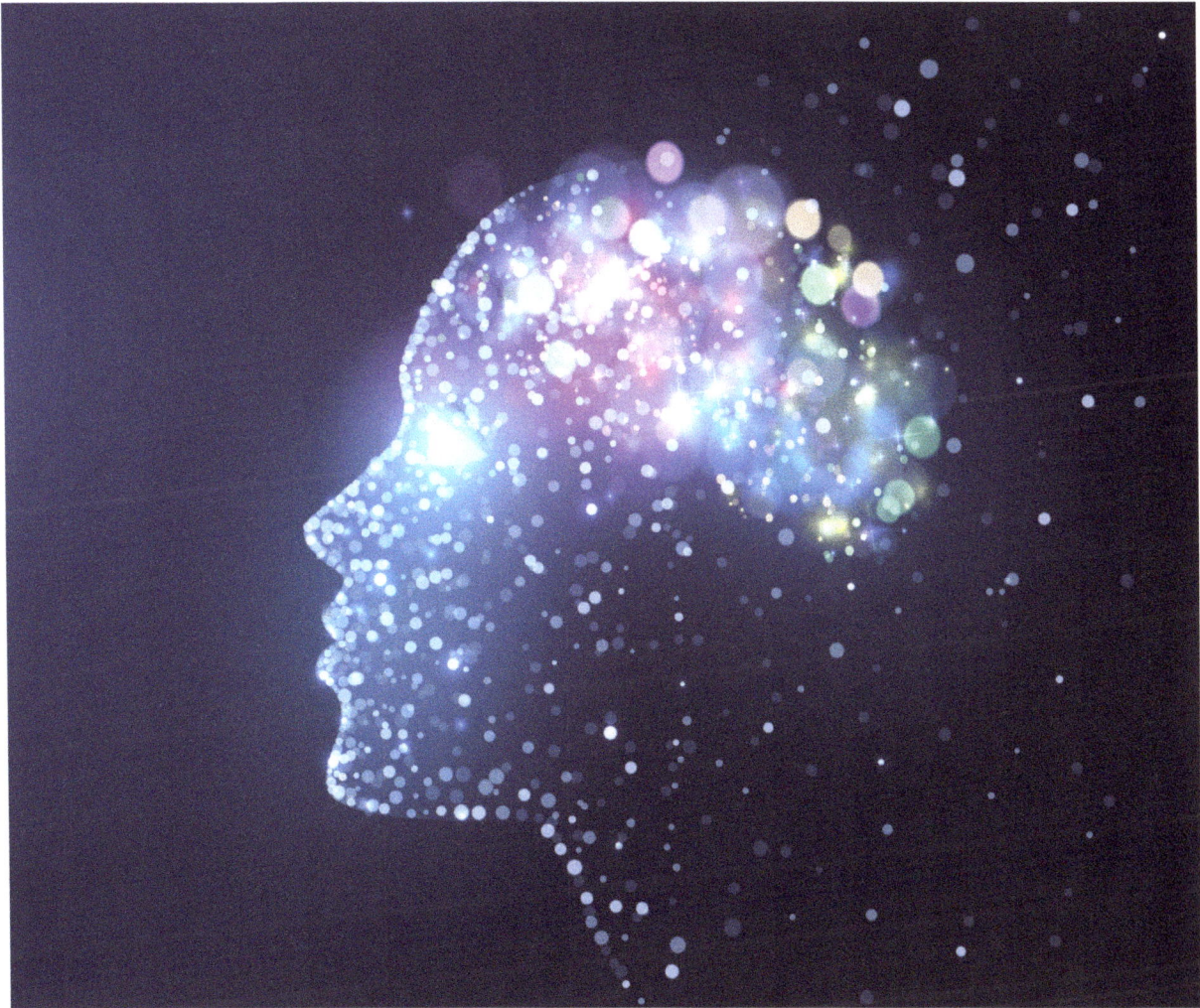

There is a bigger force at work. Some might call it a person's personality, or spirit or soul. It's definitely there, whether you can see it or not. It's like an invisible mind-cloud that is driving the body, having thoughts, making decisions, choosing movements, prompting creativity, etc.

It's the driver, or perhaps the pilot, of a person. Sure, maybe it all comes out of the brain, but try to find it. Try to touch it. It's not there — but of course it *is* there. Somewhere...?

Now we know it's "there," even if it isn't. Who's to say it's alone? In the case of an OCD person, perhaps there's another component. Maybe this other component is having input into the person's life and actions. Perhaps the driver is in pretty good control most of the time, but what if there's a back seat driver offering input, too? What if the suggestions from the back seat are not good suggestions, and the driver is distracted and struggles to ignore them? That's a good reaction, but it doesn't satisfy the back seat driver, so the suggestions are repeated endlessly.

Connect all the dots and make little boxes. And be quick!

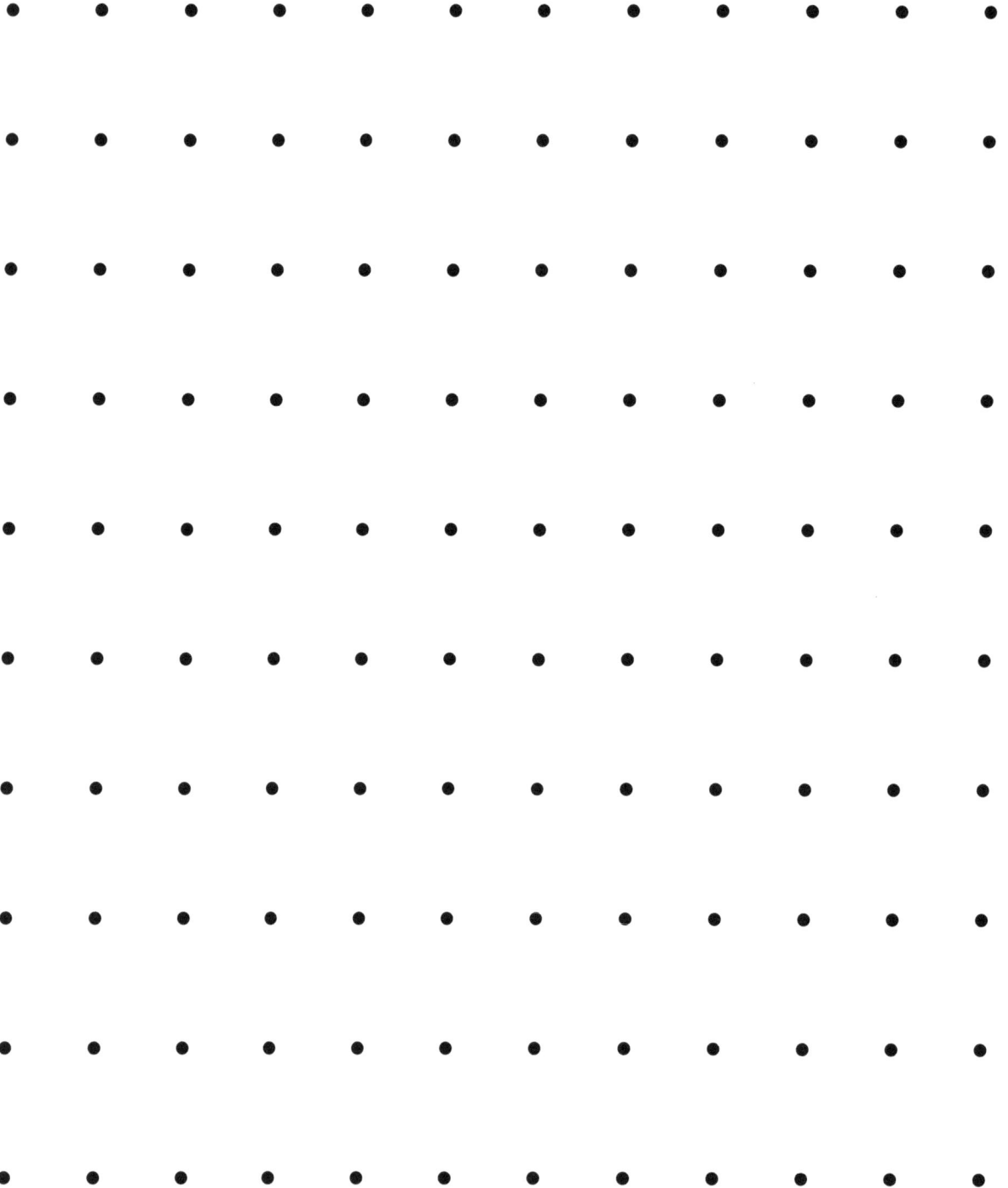

Tear out the page and then tear each box into a separate piece. Trash them all.

Maybe a better comparison is a pilot and a co-pilot. The pilot is in control of an airplane, but the co-pilot also has a set of controls. The pilot can fight to be in control, but a co-pilot can degrade the pilot's control and redirect the plane.

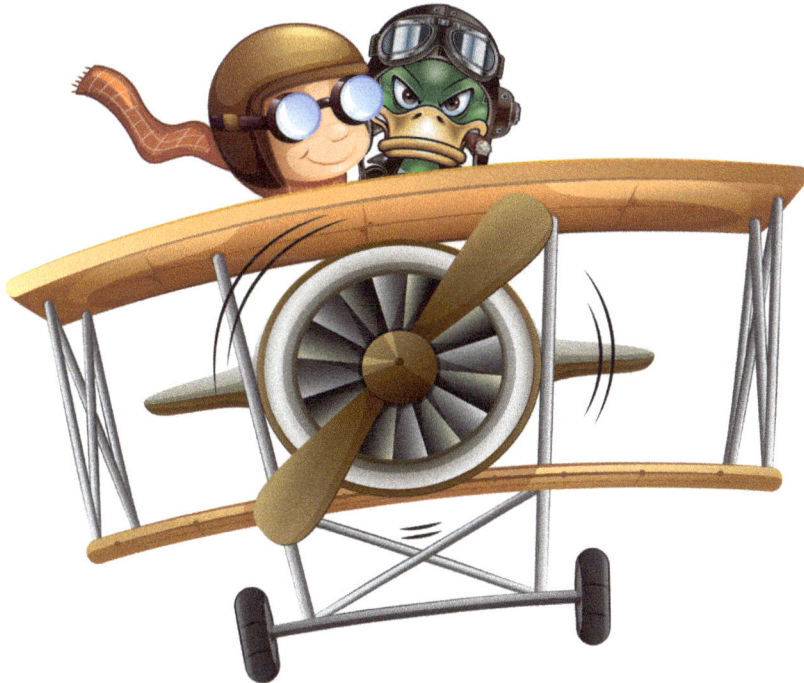

So maybe you have a pilot part of your personality that has good ideas and knows what needs to be done in your life. (Sound familiar?) But, if there's an OCD co-pilot with hands on the controls and a constant stream of bad ideas, things can deteriorate pretty quickly.

It's like having a gremlin running your life, even though there are no such things as gremlins. Maybe you'd rather think of it as some sort of OCD wizard.

Maybe you have an OCD co-pilot who is always there, whether speaking or not. The co-pilot knows the worst times to speak up with a bad idea. Sometimes it's a whisper. Sometimes it's a scream. Eventually any pilot will make a bad decision.

Maybe it just results in a single tic. An extra blink. Or an almost silent grunt. But it repeats. Over and over.

It could be a tiny little bad decision, almost nonexistent and almost without consequences. But not quite. And the co-pilot is still at work.

The co-pilot never gives up. The co-pilot never quits.

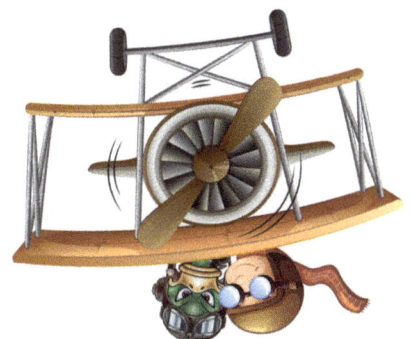

45

Tear this page out and fold it to make a paper airplane.

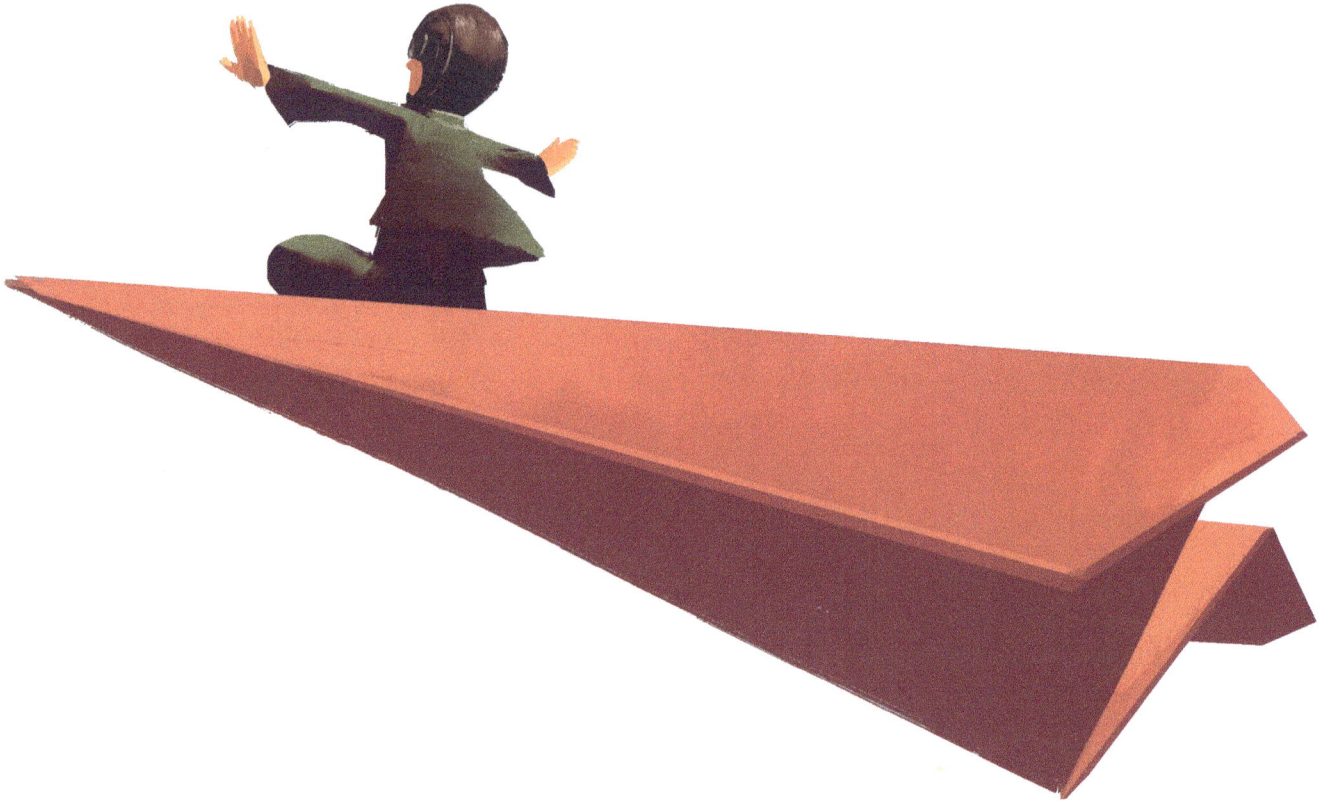

Send it flying. Walk away. Leave it!

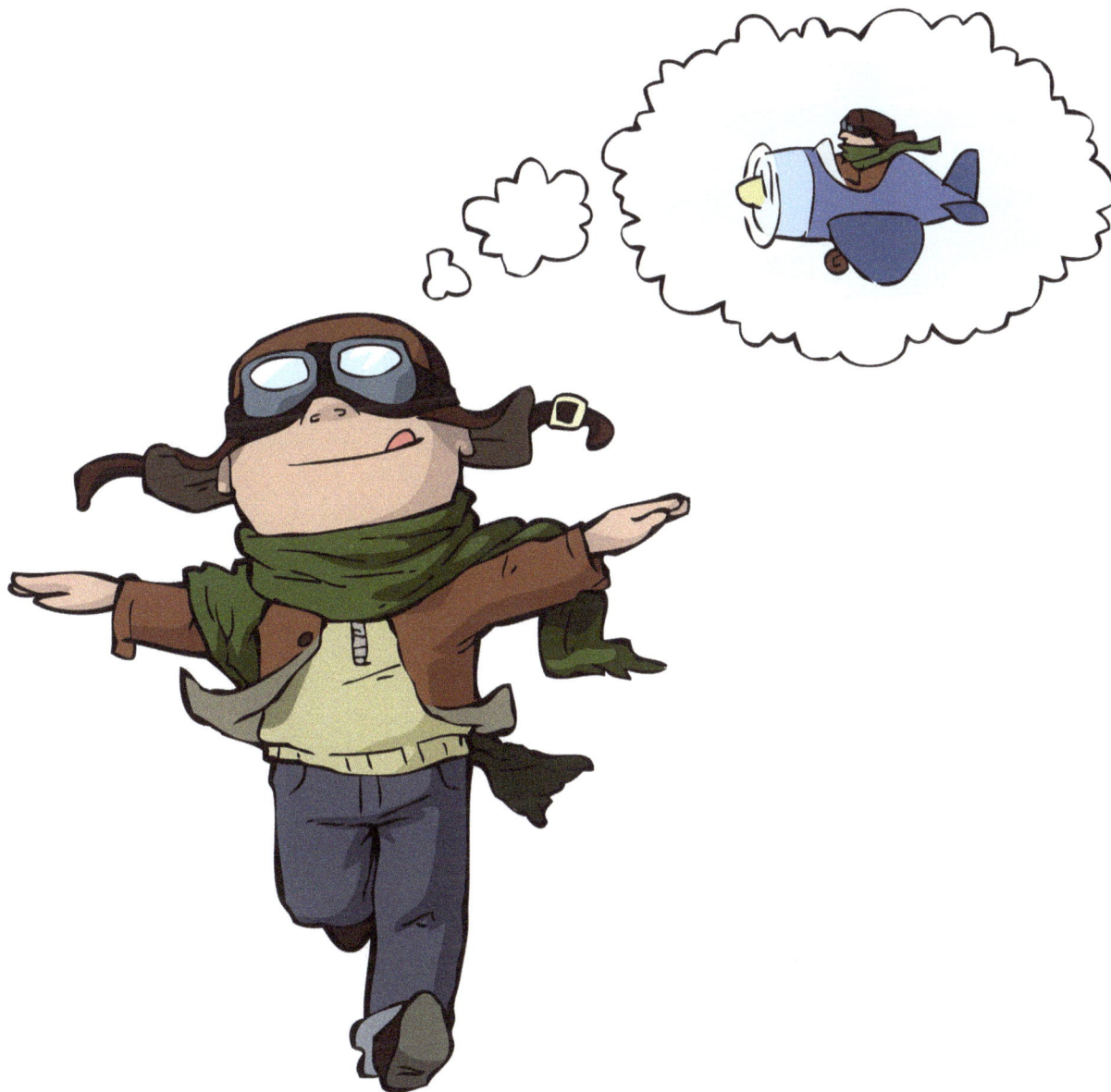

We can't see uneasy thoughts, yet we know they're there, alongside our hopes and fears. With OCD they create illogical loops of thought.

This invisible personality drives everything we do. Let the pilot fly the plane that is you. Learn to ignore the co-pilot.

Make your pilot happy.

You'll have a better flight.

Count something. Anything. Just start counting. When you finish, write the number here. Then count something else and write that number, too. Keep counting and writing the numbers until you've filled this page.

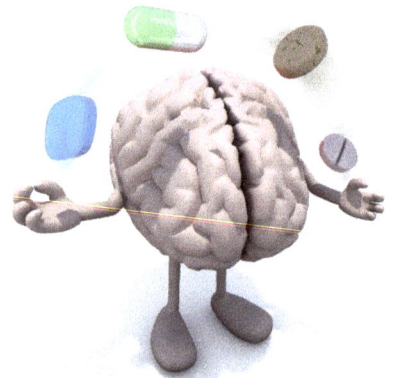

Now add up all the numbers and write the total here:_____.
Then — you guessed it — tear up the page. Count the pieces. Then stop counting.

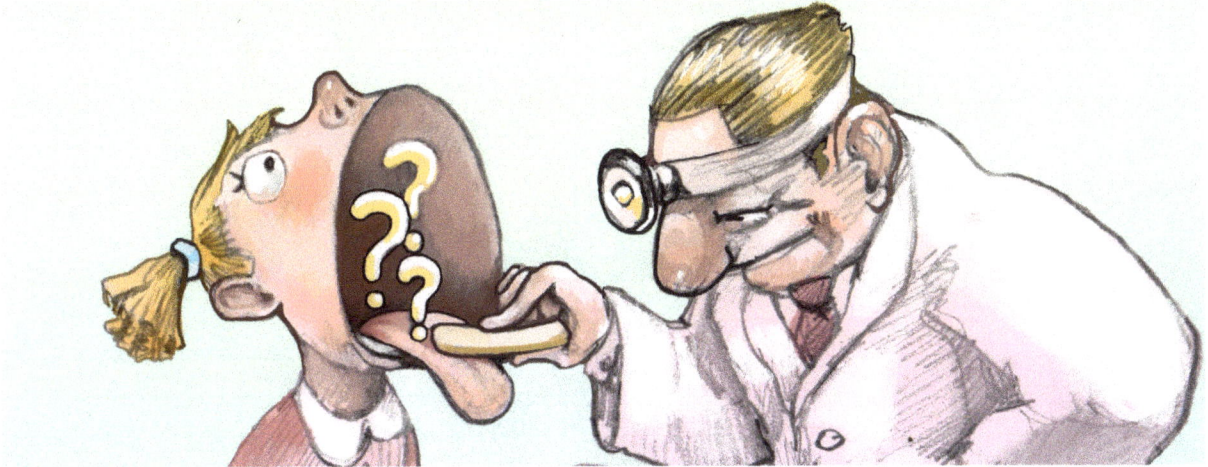

What will help?

OCD covers a large number of thoughts and actions. Some are minor annoyances, but some can be quite serious, leading to harm or injury. That makes treatment really important. There is no cure for OCD, but you can cope. You'll be fine.

Therapy can be quite helpful, offering ways to change both thoughts and behaviors. Don't be afraid to open up. You're not the first to have these thoughts and to act on them. Remember, if thinking can cause some of your problems, thinking differently can help fix them.

The most effective version is called cognitive behavior therapy, using a technique called exposure and response prevention. Under supervision, you expose yourself to your obsessions and then prevent yourself from a compulsion response.

There are also medicines that can be effective, especially helping with tics. Drugs are not a cure, but they can help with control.

There are even surgical techniques that are sometimes being used. The important thing is to get some help in whatever way is available to you.

Since OCD is stress inducing, relaxation is always good — try yoga, meditation, and massage. Sometimes a good laugh can help you relax. Sleep can help, too, as can physical activity. Also, a good diet can help to keep blood sugar levels normal.

New treatments are being developed as well, including techniques that include magnetic and/or electrical stimulation. Currently most of these are for more serious cases and can potentially have unwelcome side effects. But, it means there's hope and there's progress. Stay tuned....

Make a List - Any List

1. _____	41. _____
2. _____	42. _____
3. _____	43. _____
4. _____	44. _____
5. _____	45. _____
6. _____	46. _____
7. _____	47. _____
8. _____	48. _____
9. _____	49. _____
10. _____	50. _____
11. _____	51. _____
12. _____	52. _____
13. _____	53. _____
14. _____	54. _____
15. _____	55. _____
16. _____	56. _____
17. _____	57. _____
18. _____	58. _____
19. _____	59. _____
20. _____	60. _____
21. _____	61. _____
22. _____	62. _____
23. _____	63. _____
24. _____	64. _____
25. _____	65. _____
26. _____	66. _____
27. _____	67. _____
28. _____	68. _____
29. _____	69. _____
30. _____	70. _____
31. _____	71. _____
32. _____	72. _____
33. _____	73. _____
34. _____	74. _____
35. _____	75. _____
36. _____	76. _____
37. _____	77. _____
38. _____	78. _____
39. _____	79. _____
40. _____	80. _____

Now tear up the list and throw it away. Stop making lists.

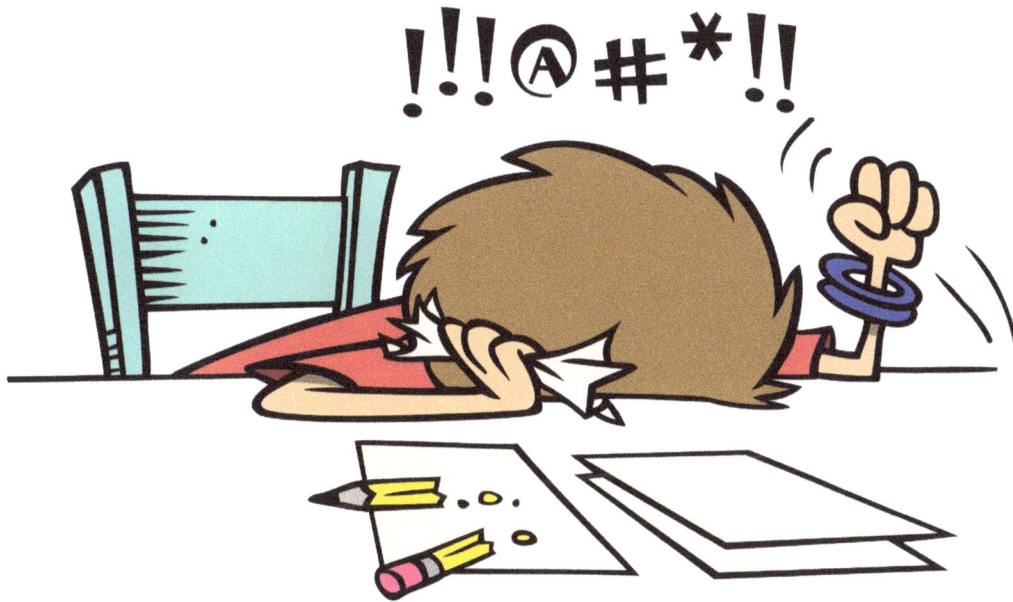

What Can I Do?

Ask for help.

Start with your parents.

Talk to your teacher.

Visit your doctor.

Here's an idea.

If you feel a familiar obsession coming on, instead of giving in and doing whatever you feel compelled to do — *do something else! Distract yourself.*

It could be anything. Go for a walk. Read a book. Make a sandwich. Do your homework. Sing a song. Or dance. When you finish that, if the compulsion is still there, find something else to do. Keep going. Stay busy.

Show your compulsions that you know they aren't justified. Confront your OCD. Can your obsessive fears come true? No!

But — they will only go away if you don't give in. Even if it's hard, keep fighting. They have just become a habit. Challenge your fears.

And get help. We all want help, but we don't want to ask for it. Ask!

WRITE THE WORST TEN THINGS YOU HATE ABOUT OCD.
(You were supposed to stop making lists!)

1.
2.
3.
4.
5.
6.
7.
8.
9.
10.
11.
12.
13.
14.
15.
16.
17.
18.
19.
20.
21.
22.
23.
24.
25.
26.
27.
28.
29.
30.
31.
32.
33.
34.
35.
36.
37.
38.
39.
40. *Tear out this page and make ten copies. Fold them neatly and throw them away.*
41.
42.

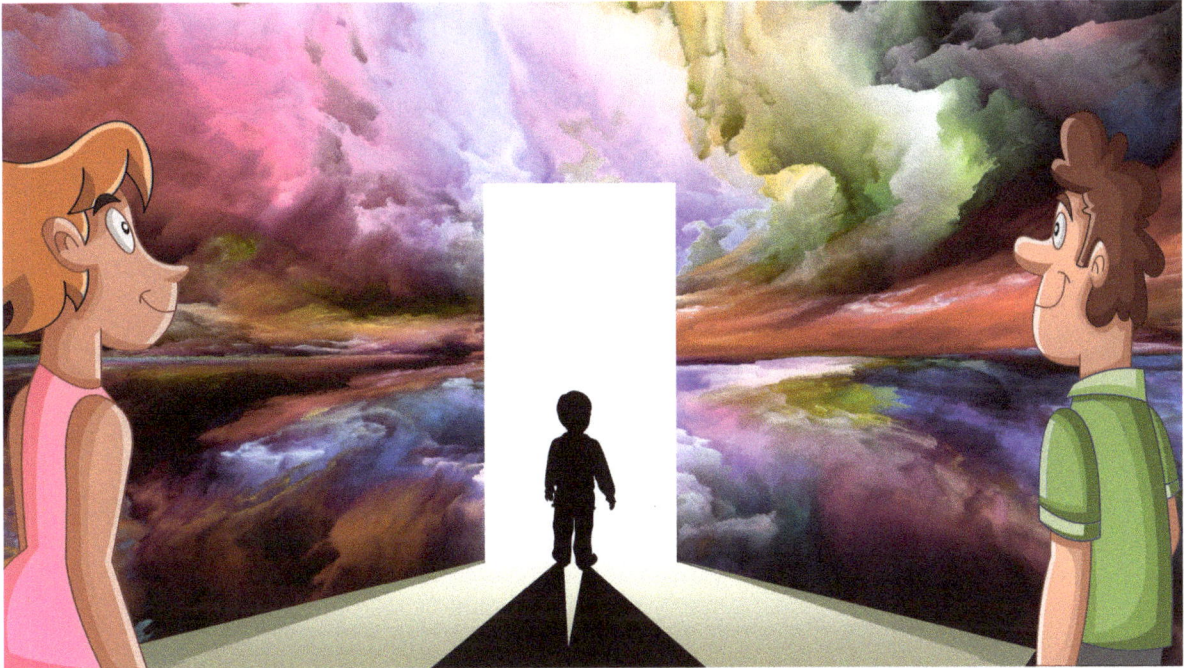

Parents

At some point your parents are going to notice.

And, they're going to ask you why you're doing whatever it is you're doing.

Instead of being annoyed and denying that anything is going on, perhaps that would be a good time to ask them to get you some help.

Your parents probably won't know exactly what to do, but they are better equipped to find someone who can offer some help.

It may start with a trip to a doctor. Even though most physicians are not experts in the OCD field, your doctor should be able to recommend someone who can help. Ask about a therapist who has experience treating OCD.

It may take several different visits before you find a solution that works for you (everybody's different), but it's important to get some control early, before everything gets more complicated.

And, don't be embarrassed. Just get help.

Stop washing your hands!

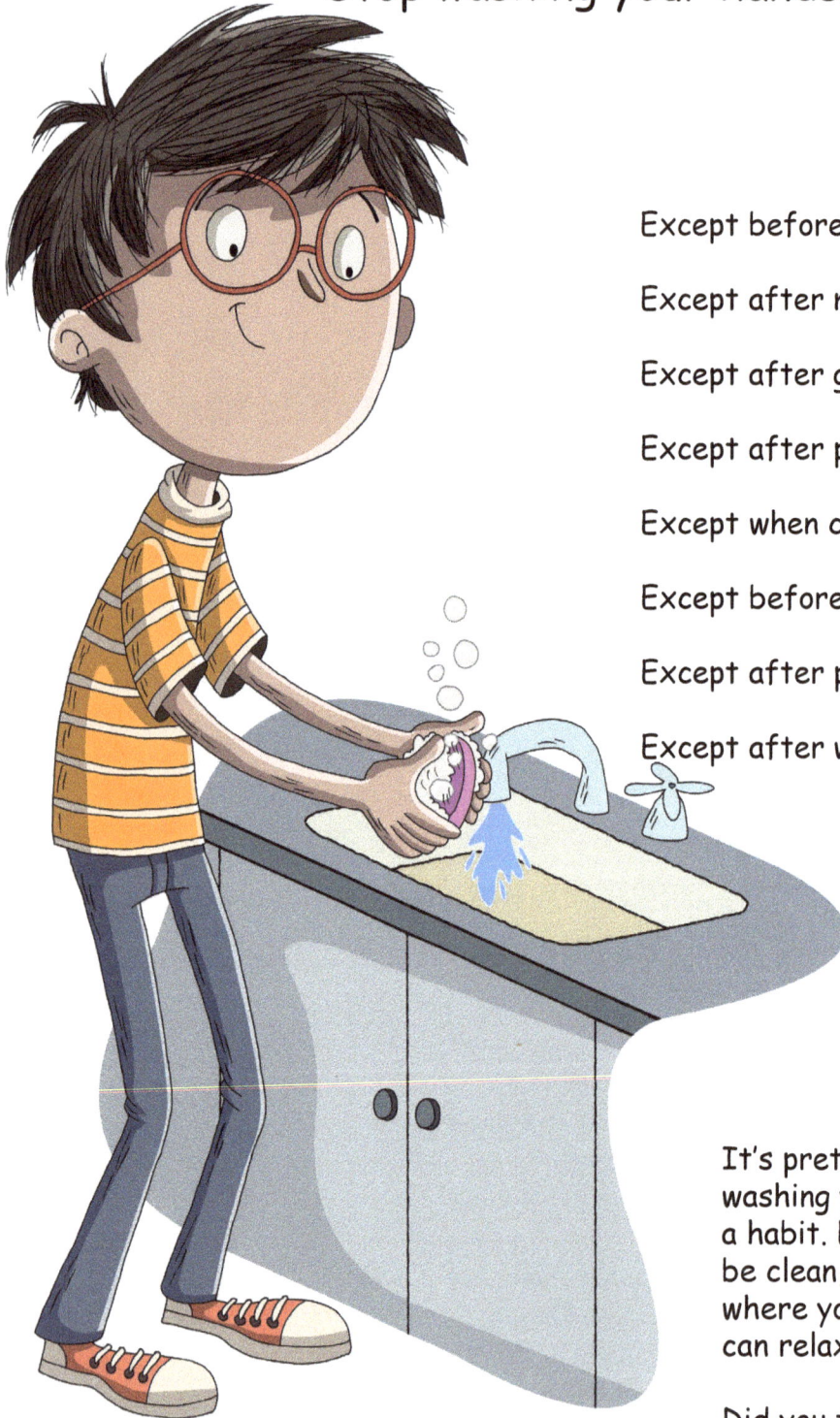

Except before meals.

Except after meals.

Except after going to the bathroom.

Except after playing with animals.

Except when cleaning up after pets.

Except before preparing food.

Except after preparing food.

Except after working at dirty jobs.

It's pretty easy to see how washing your hands can become a habit. Everyone wants you to be clean, but there's a point where you *are* clean, and you can relax.

Did you turn off the water?

Use your unwashed hands to tear this page out and tear it into little pieces.

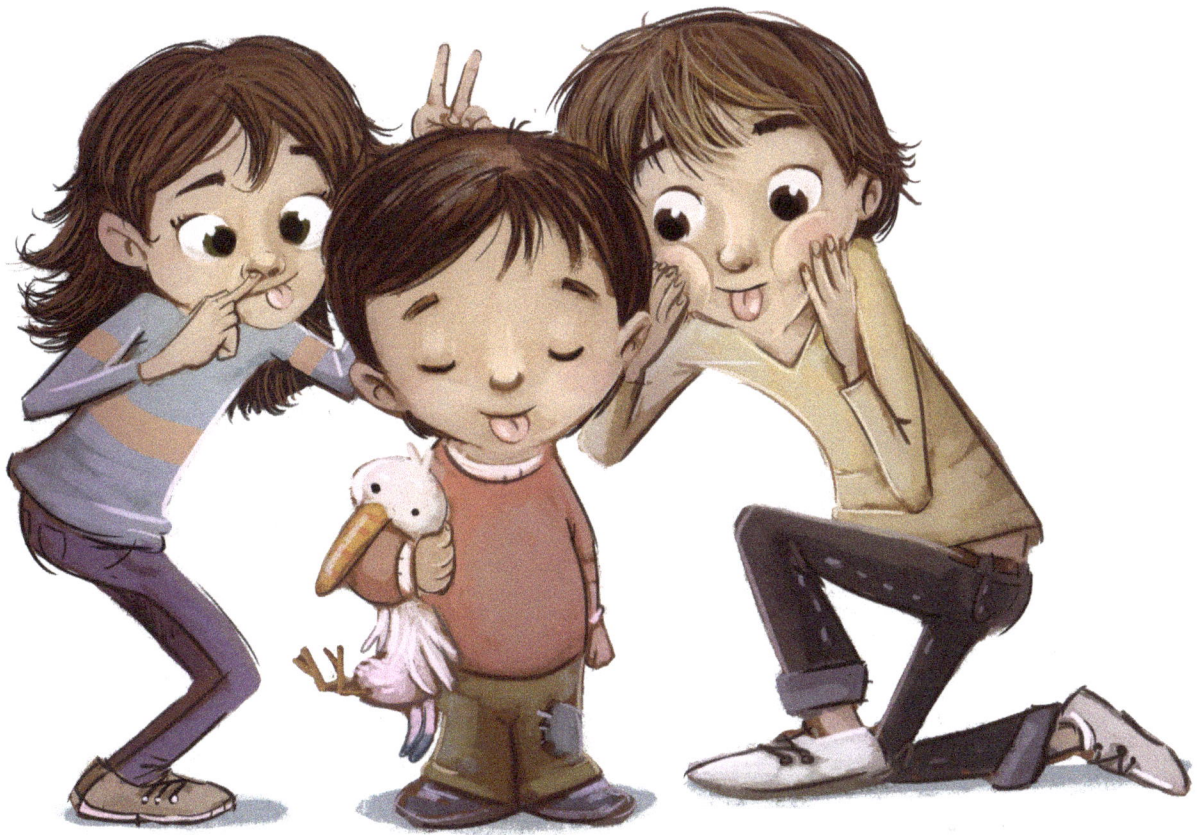

Getting Teased?

When it comes to kids (and some adults) anything different quickly becomes the subject of ridicule.

You may hear it, or it may all be behind your back.

This is unfortunate and unhelpful. There is no easy answer to this kind of behavior, especially when OCD already comes with lots of doubts and feelings of inferiority. You're not inferior! You're just going to have to be strong.

There is a rare form of teasing that is meant to be friendly and hopes to call attention to your behavior in a helpful way — hopefully to lead to some positive action on your part. But it's still teasing and it still hurts.

Bullying is never an easy thing to deal with, but it says more about the bully than it does you. Talk to your therapist or counselor.

You have probably been routinely checking page numbers, but this page doesn't have a correct page number. Or does it? What should it be? Don't check other pages for hints!

Tear it out and rip it up.

239 - 24 - 15 - 7 - 19 - 21C - 13 - 56 - 39 - 42 - 56 - 12 - 519 - 2 -319

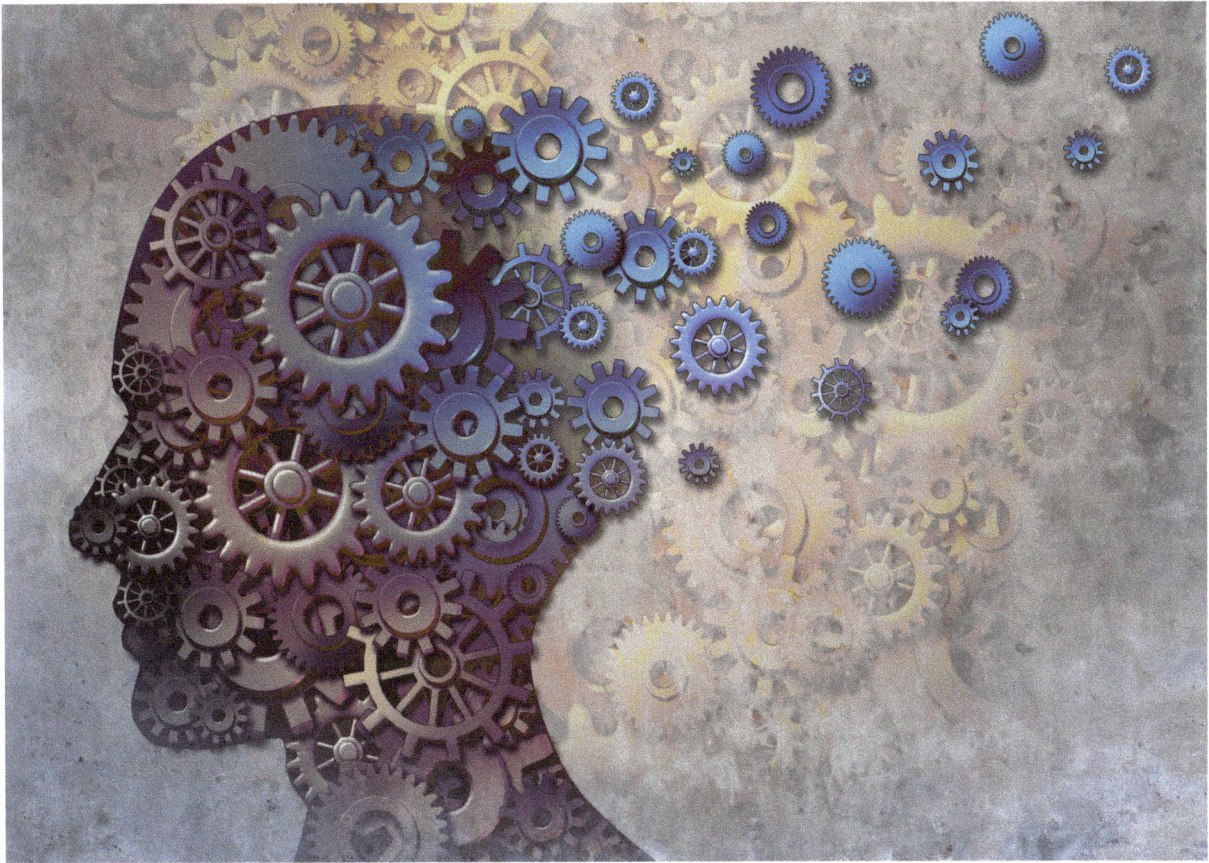

Other Related Problems

In addition to OCD, you can also have some of the exact same symptoms and behaviors as other disorders.

OCD tics and noises are just like Tourette's Syndrome. Fear of leaving the house is like agouraphobia. There are eating disorders — obsessions with food — such as binge eating, anorexia nervosa, and bulimia.

Depression, attention deficit/hyperactivity disorder (ADHD), phobias, bipolar disorder, post-traumatic stress disorder (PTSD), body dysmorphic disorder (fear of imagined ugliness), and panic attacks are common OCD issues, and they are disorders of their own, as well.

Adding to the confusion, there is something called Obsessive Compulsive Personality Disorder (OCPD) that is often and easily confused with OCD. In particular, it deals with perfectionism and rigid fixations with lists and rules.

It's similar, but different. (Your therapist can explain.)

Do not look at this page number!

Do not tear out this page! Unless you think of a monkey.

What was it you were not supposed to think of? Oh. Right. Then tear it out.

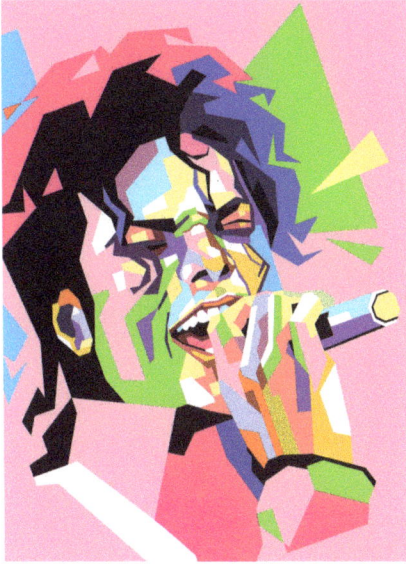

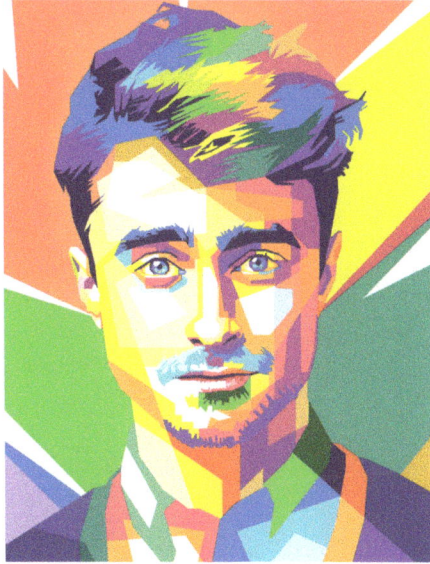

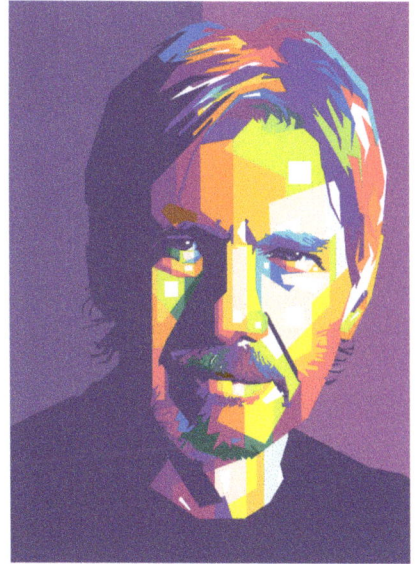

Having OCD is not the end of the world.

There are plenty of people dealing with OCD besides you, and you've probably known some of them whether you knew it or not. (You've definitely noticed someone with a tic or habit.)

Many have gone on to great success despite their OCD. You can do the same.

Some of the people on this list have talked openly about their struggle with OCD: David Beckham, Katy Perry, Leonardo DiCaprio, Lena Dunham, Howard Stern, Justin Timberlake, Howie Mandel, Jessica Alba, Daniel Radcliffe, Charlize Theron, Cameron Diaz, Megan Fox, Billy Bob Thornton, Julianne Moore, Charlie Sheen, Harrison Ford, Jennifer Love Hewitt, Dan Aykroyd, Emily Lloyd, Martin Scorsese, Michael Jackson, Penelope Cruz, Roseanne Barr, Woody Allen, Alec Baldwin, Warren Zevon, Alanis Morissette, and Donald Trump.

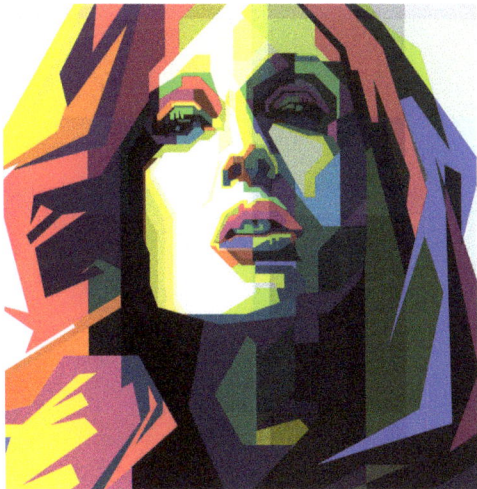

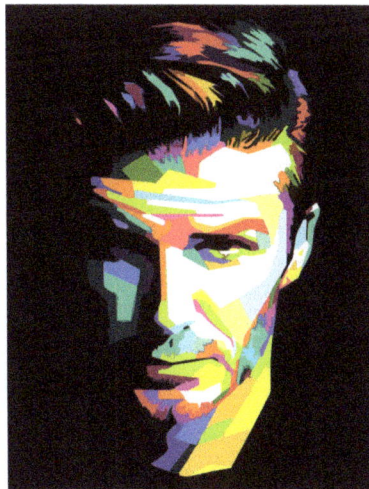

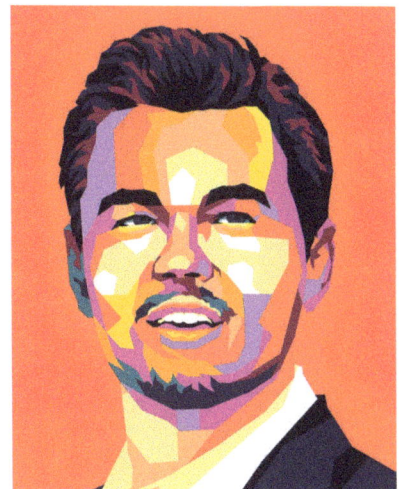

This page is out of order. It should have been the next page. Tear it out and put it after the next page.

Charles Darwin

Bill Gates

Stephen Hawking

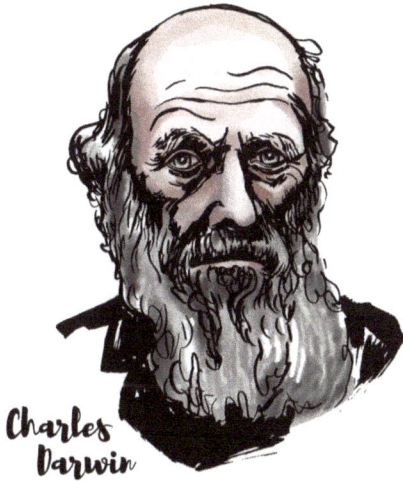

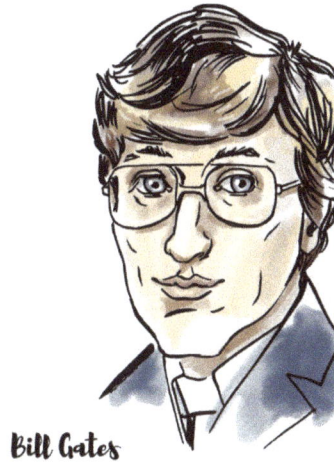

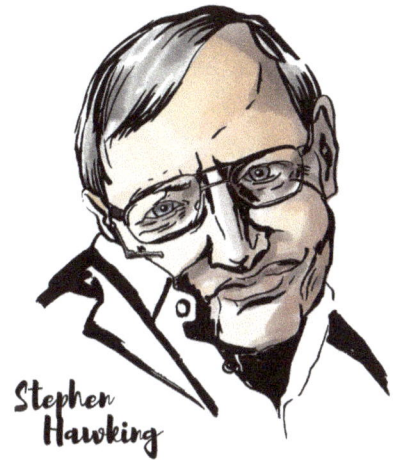

There are legendary people down through the ages who we believe, in hindsight, probably had OCD.

Experts have reviewed stories, evidence, and behaviors of famous people throughout history and evaluated them for OCD tendencies. There's no way to actually be certain, but the symptoms are pretty clear and strongly suggest OCD.

These include some of our greatest minds, with many notable successes:

Nicola Tesla, Howard Hughes, Frank Sinatra, Martin Luther, Charles Darwin, John Bunyan, Dr. Samuel Johnson, Albert Einstein, Ludwig van Beethoven, Michaelangelo, Charles Dickens, Cole Porter, Andrew Kehoe, Gerald Kaufman, Marcel Proust, Sir Winston Churchill, Stanley Kubrick, Andy Warhol, Marie Curie, Issac Newton, Isaac Asimov, Stephen Hawking, Bill Gates, and Steve Jobs.

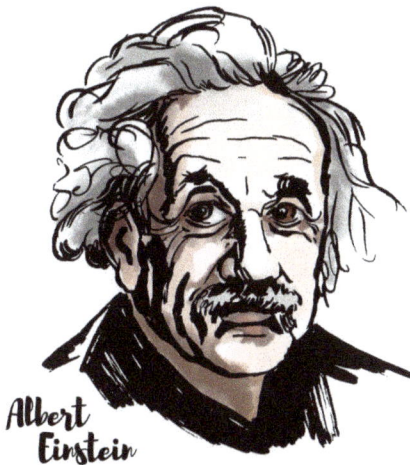

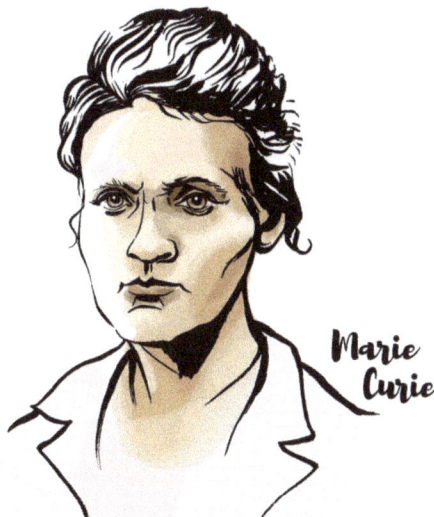

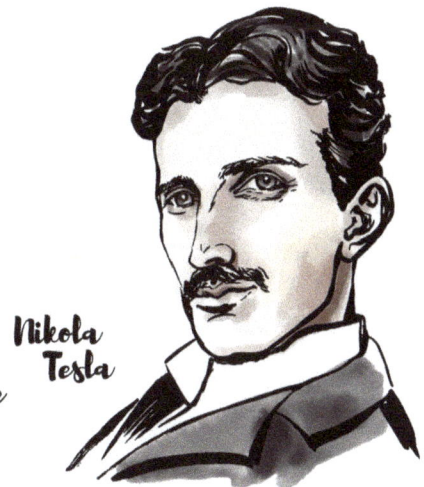

Albert Einstein

Marie Curie

Nikola Tesla

Oh, great. Now this page is out of order. Tear it out and put it after the last page that you tore out and put after this one. And keep doing it until you get it right.

Are you dizzy yet? Throw both pages away, but not until they're in the right order.

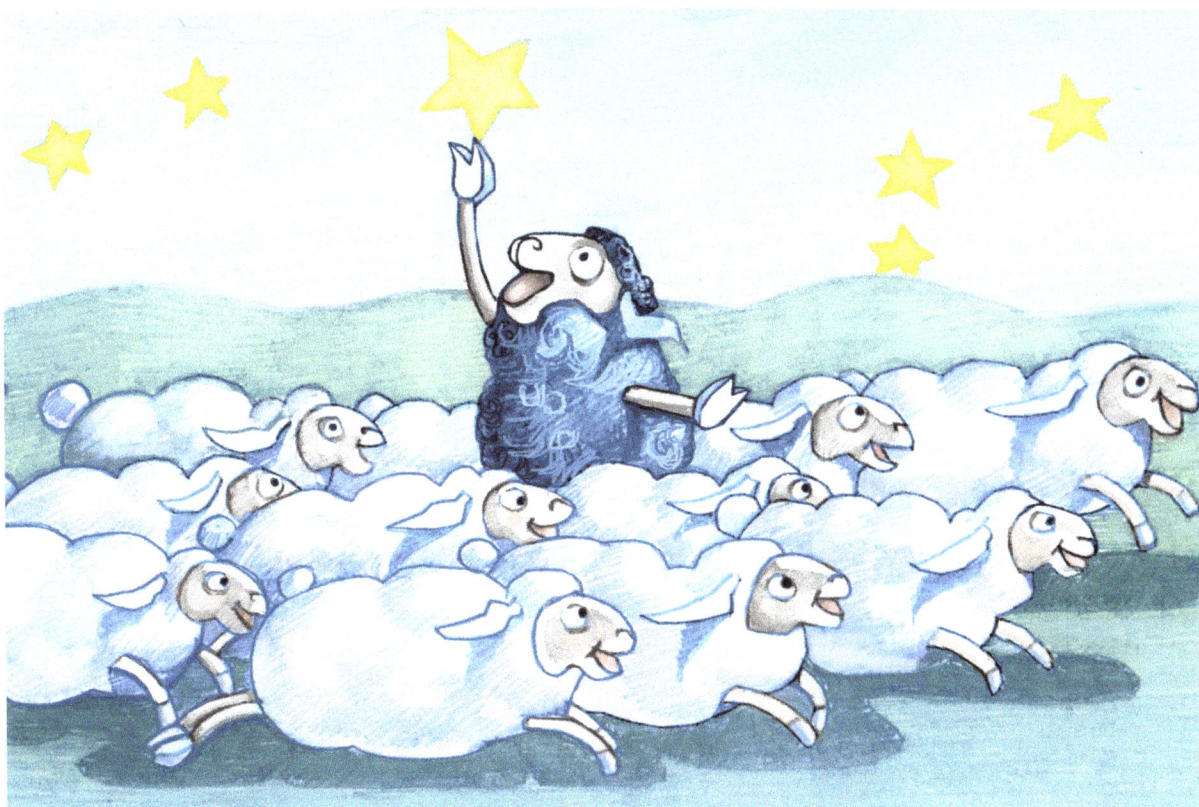

Be Bold

Don't be afraid of OCD. It can definitely cause problems in your day-to-day life, but you can tame it, and you can still do great things.

As you've seen here, there have been many successful people who have lived with OCD, but did not let it stop them. You're going to be one of those people.

You're probably good at brainstorming and you're empathetic. And, you're good at time management, with superior attention to detail. You meet deadlines, too, typically bringing a hyperfocus to tasks, with an increased level of perseverance.

You don't have to become an inventor or a scientist or a famous actor or singer to be successful (but you might). There are many different paths to success.

Some people call OCD their Superpower, but it's not that easy. OCD is more of a tool. When used properly, along with plenty of hard work, the OCD tool can help you achieve great results

You're going to find your own path to deal with OCD. You're going to be happy.

The next page is the end. But if you're truly OCD you'll keep going. And going. And going. And going....

So tear this page out very carefully. In fact, you should use scissors. Then chop it into as many pieces as you can. Then count them. And stack them. Then stop doing all this.

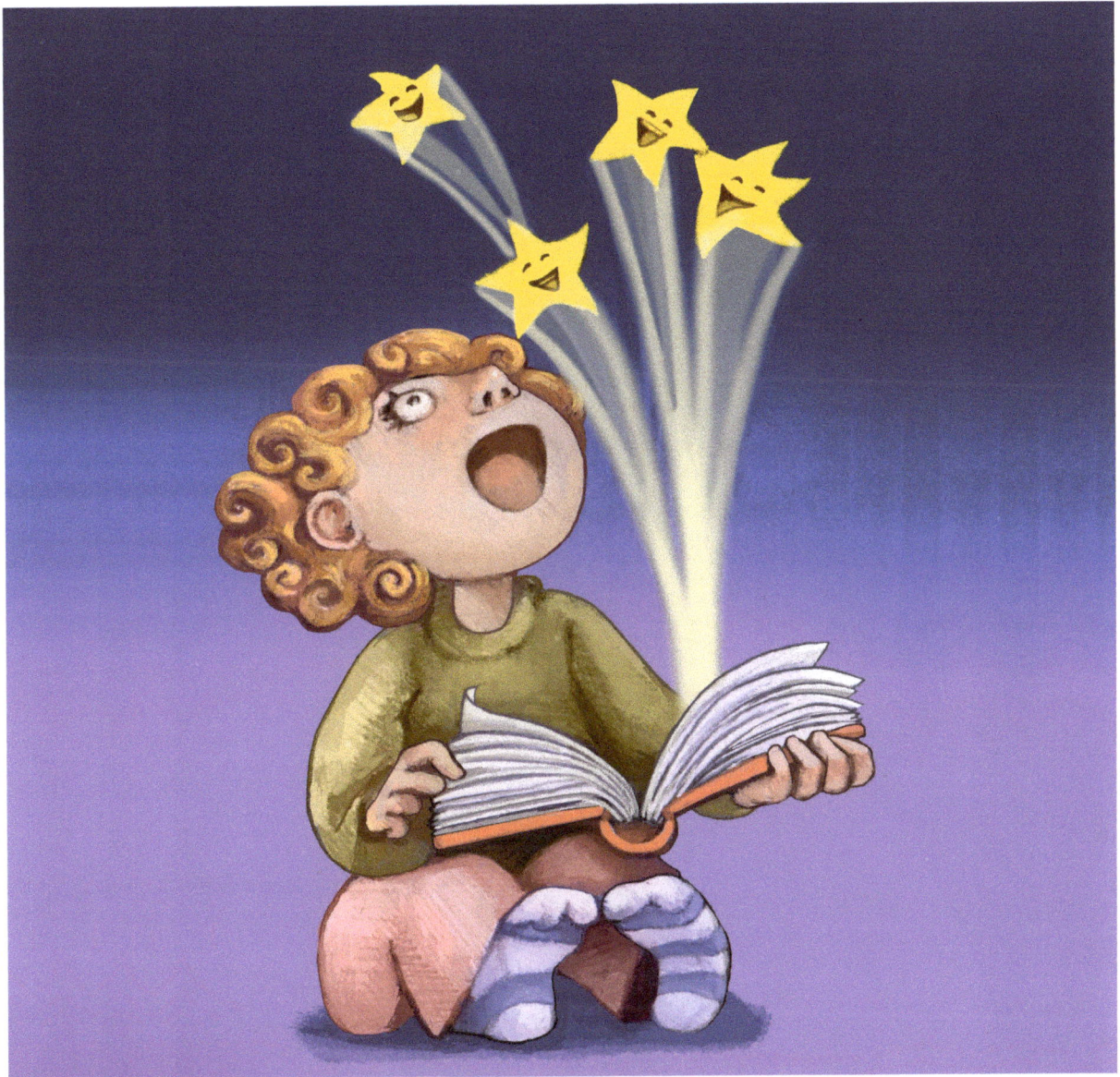

It's been said that one aspect of OCD can be increased creativity, as shown by the considerable number of successful people with OCD.

So now it's time for you to turn some of that creativity into solving the problems that come with OCD. You can do it. Celebrate your OCD!

You're going to find success. And happiness!

THE END

DO NOT TEAR THIS PAGE OUT!!!!

This is the test of will and determination that is the first step out of your OCD. (The next step is to get professional help.)

Of course if you need to re-read the earlier pages you'll probably want another copy since this one is now ruined. (Good for you!)

You should hurry because this was a precious First Edition and one of the last copies. It would have been a collector's item, worth a fortune.

There *might* be one copy left. Maybe. If you're lucky, you can find the very last undestroyed copy of this wonderful book at *www.cosworthpublishing.com*.

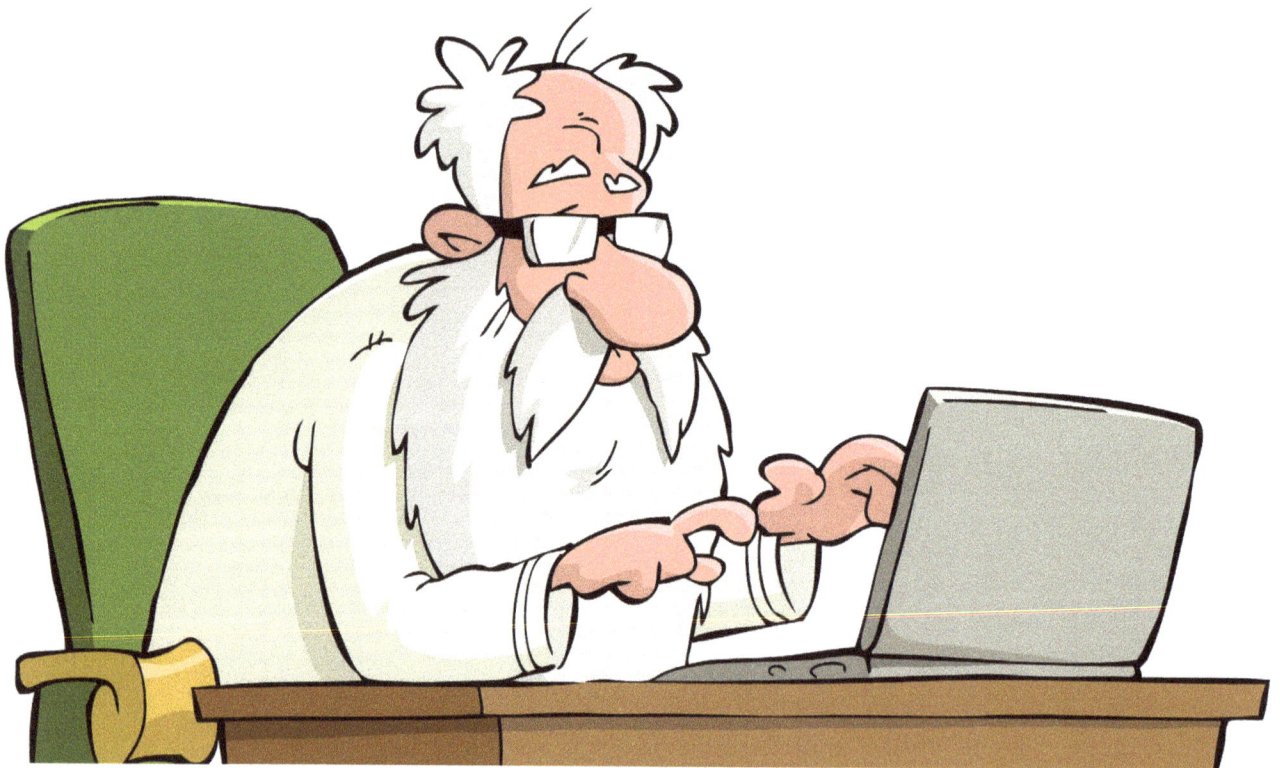

About the Author

Jimmy Huston wrote this book wrote this book wrote this book. He has just enough OCD stuff going on that it forced him to finish it, but not enough to make him clean his room clean his room clean his room. He lives in Woodland Hills, California, with his wife and dog, who have both just about had enough.

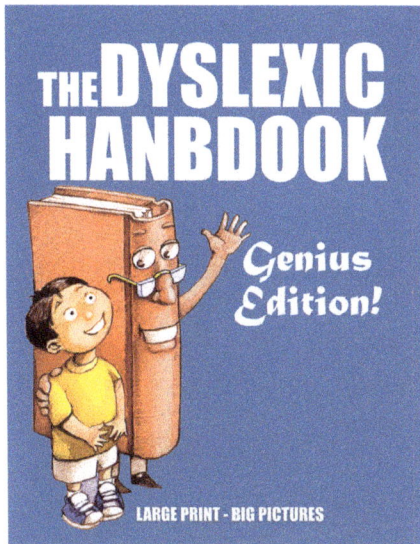

THE DYSLEXIC HANBDOOK

Genius Edition!

LARGE PRINT - BIG PICTURES

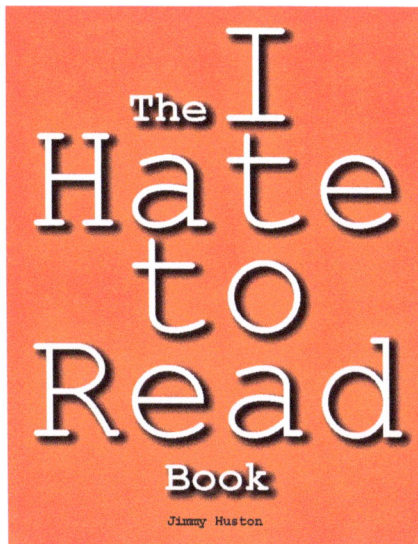

The I Hate to Read Book

Jimmy Huston

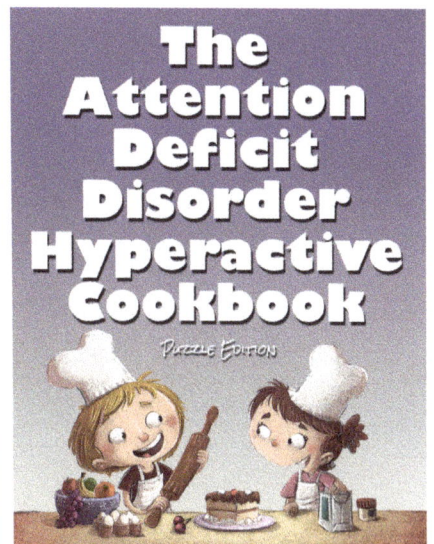

The Attention Deficit Disorder Hyperactive Cookbook

Puzzle Edition

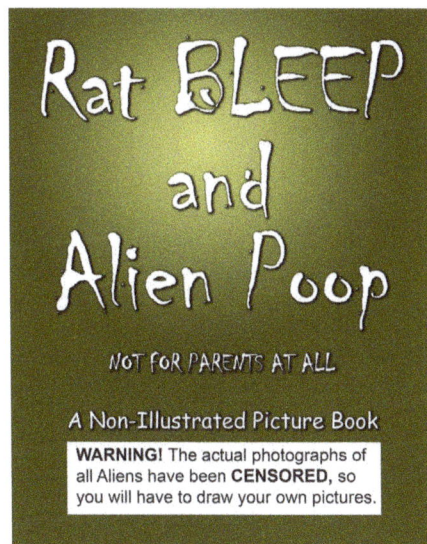

Rat BLEEP and Alien Poop

NOT FOR PARENTS AT ALL

A Non-Illustrated Picture Book

WARNING! The actual photographs of all Aliens have been **CENSORED**, so you will have to draw your own pictures.

Non-Cookbooks from Cosworth Publishing

www.cosworthpublishing.com

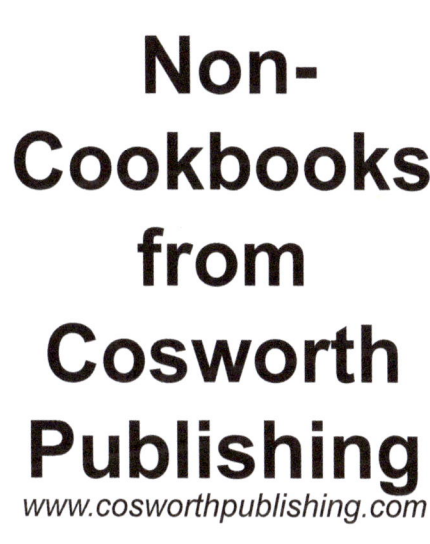

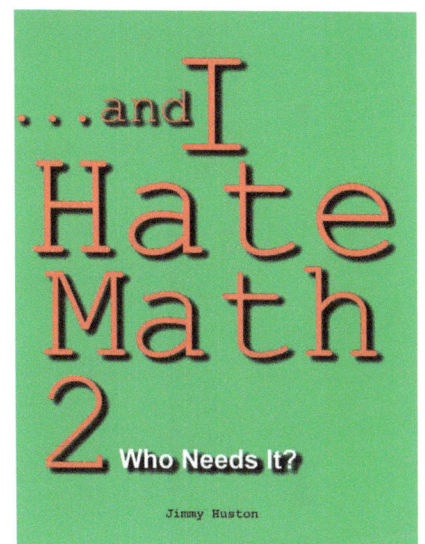

...and I Hate Math 2

Who Needs It?

Jimmy Huston

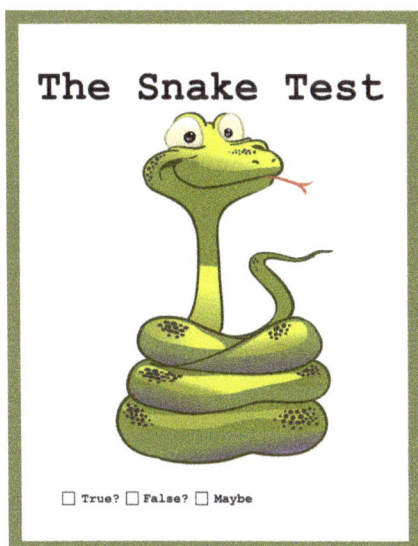

The Snake Test

☐ True? ☐ False? ☐ Maybe

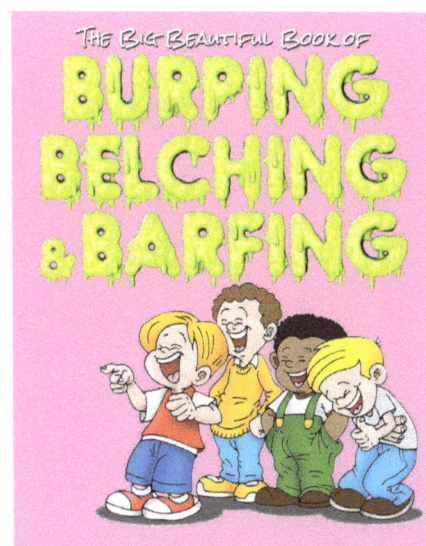

THE BIG BEAUTIFUL BOOK OF BURPING BELCHING & BARFING

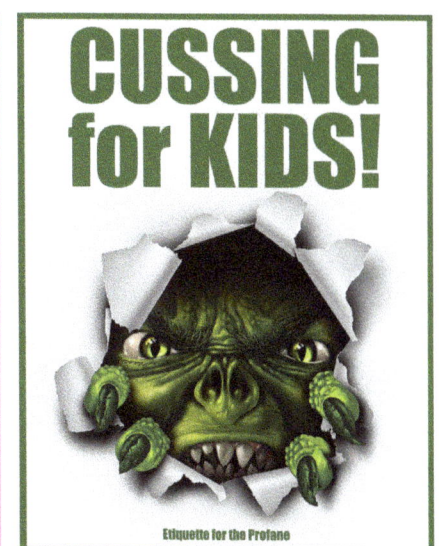

CUSSING for KIDS!

Etiquette for the Profane

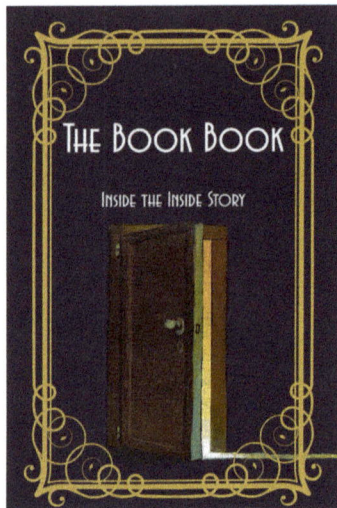

The Book Book

INSIDE THE INSIDE STORY

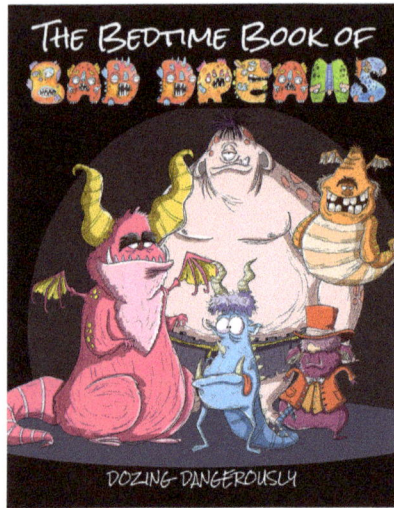

THE BEDTIME BOOK OF **BAD DREAMS**

DOZING DANGEROUSLY

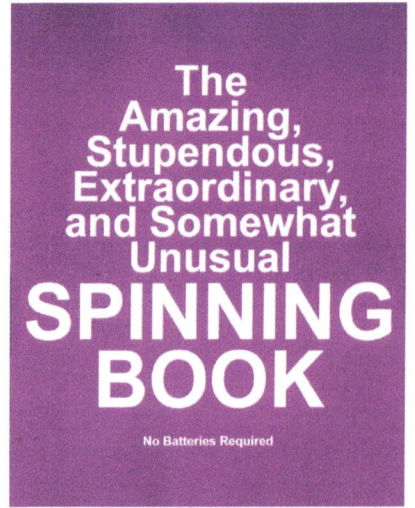

The Amazing, Stupendous, Extraordinary, and Somewhat Unusual SPINNING BOOK

No Batteries Required

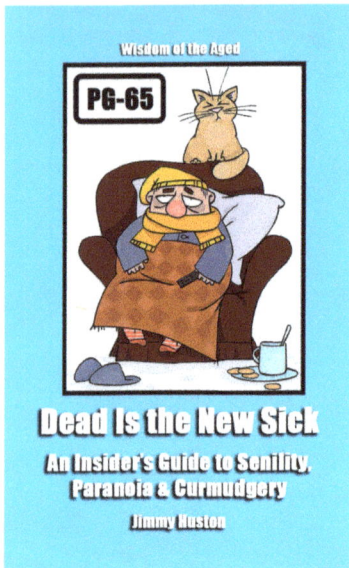

Wisdom of the Aged

PG-65

Dead Is the New Sick

An Insider's Guide to Senility, Paranoia & Curmudgery

Jimmy Huston

Non-Cookbooks from Cosworth Publishing

www.cosworthpublishing.com

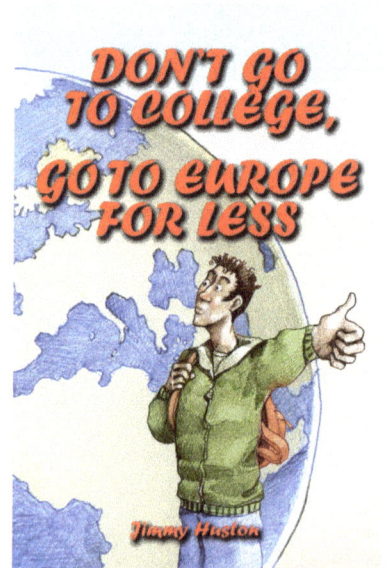

DON'T GO TO COLLEGE, GO TO EUROPE FOR LESS

Jimmy Huston

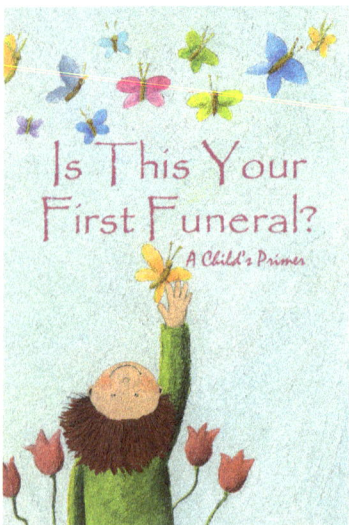

Is This Your First Funeral? A Child's Primer

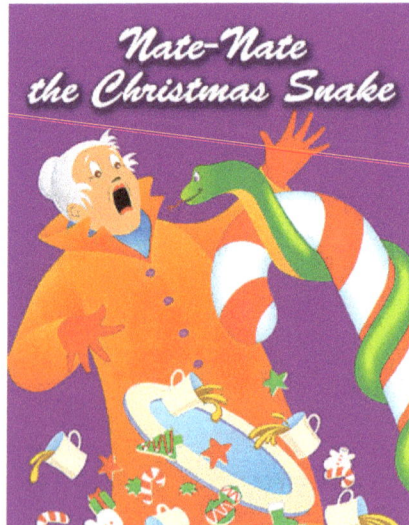

Nate-Nate the Christmas Snake

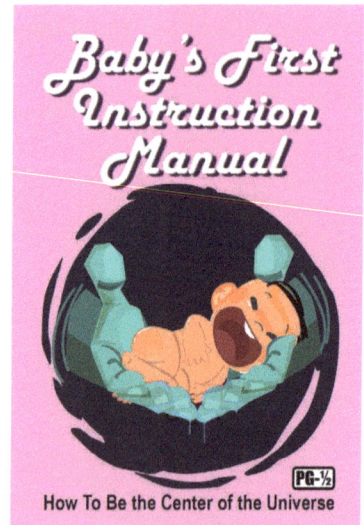

Baby's First Instruction Manual

PG-½

How To Be the Center of the Universe

Find it wherever good books are dreaded.

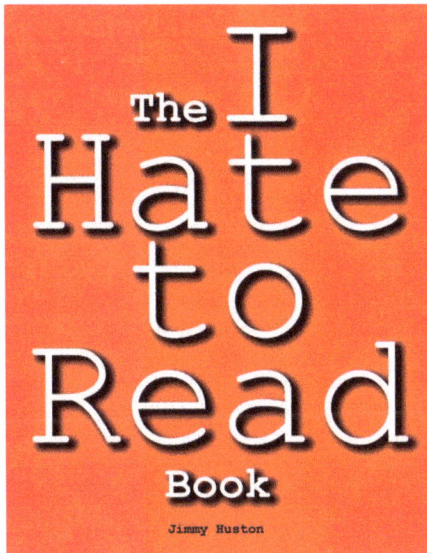

The I Hate to Read Book
Jimmy Huston

If you're reading this, you will not like this book. It's not for you.

This book is for all the people who are *not* reading this.

They won't like it either, but it's short.

They'll like that.

"I didn't actually read this book. If I had, I would have loved it — but I never will."
Billy

"'Hate' isn't a strong enough word for me. I loathe reading. I don't even like looking at pictures — which there are none of."
Wally

"This isn't what I wrote about this stupid book."
Zane

"This is an excellent coffee table book, if your coffee table hates to read."
Solomon

"This book made my teacher cry."
David

"My son loved this book. He said it was delicious."
Mr. Jones

"THIS BOOK IS SO DUMB THAT I COULD'VE WRITTEN IT."
Jimmy

www.i-hate-to-read.com

How to Write This Book!

You're going to be the author.

_____
(Write your name here.)

THE OCD FUNBOOK

REALLY?

Why Can't Mommy Spend More Time with Me?

SO YOU REALLY WANT A DOG?
A Kid's Guide to Getting a Dog

Learn What You Need to Know to Show Your Parents You're Ready

Lynn Mills

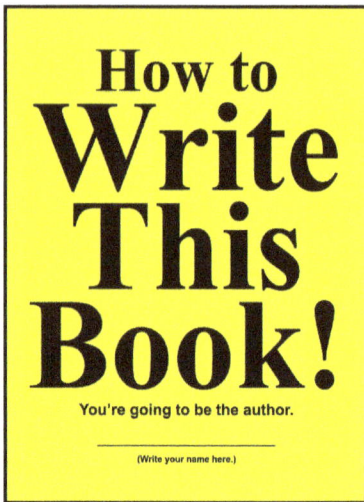

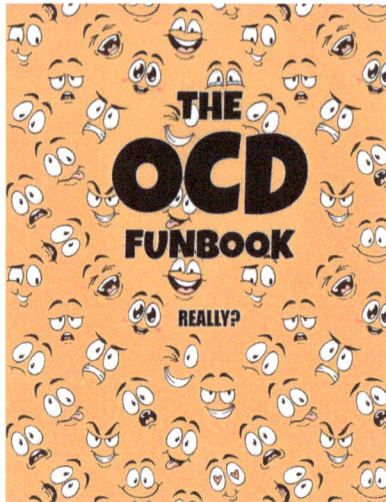

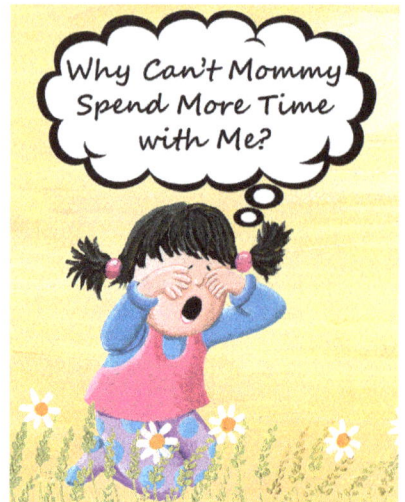

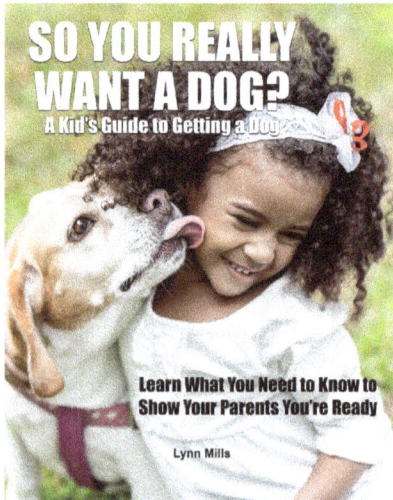

More Books from Cosworth Publishing
www.cosworthpublishing.com

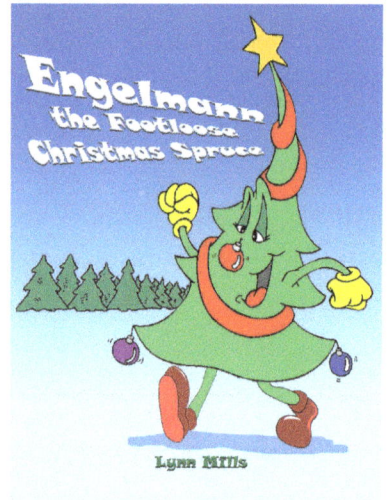

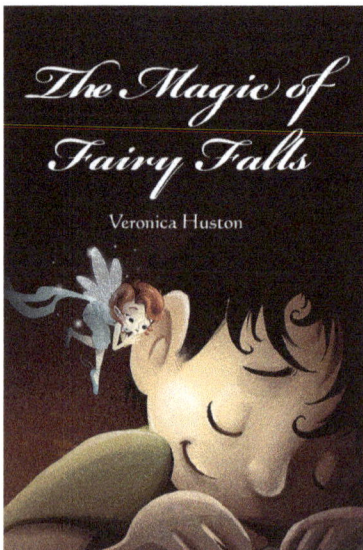

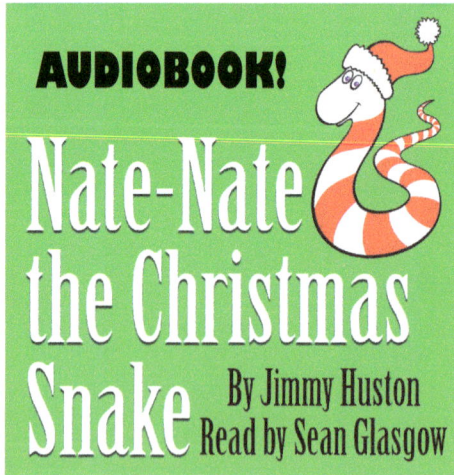

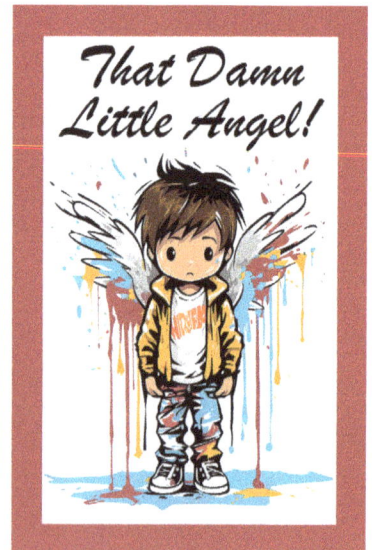

Engelmann the Footloose Christmas Spruce

Lynn Mills

The Magic of Fairy Falls
Veronica Huston

AUDIOBOOK!
Nate-Nate the Christmas Snake
By Jimmy Huston
Read by Sean Glasgow

That Damn Little Angel!

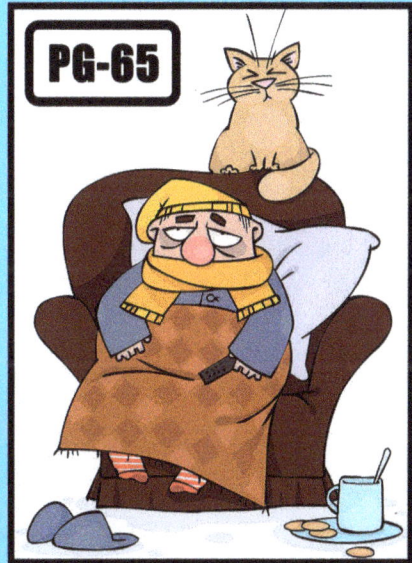

Dead Is the New Sick
An Insider's Guide to Senility, Paranoia, & Curmudgery

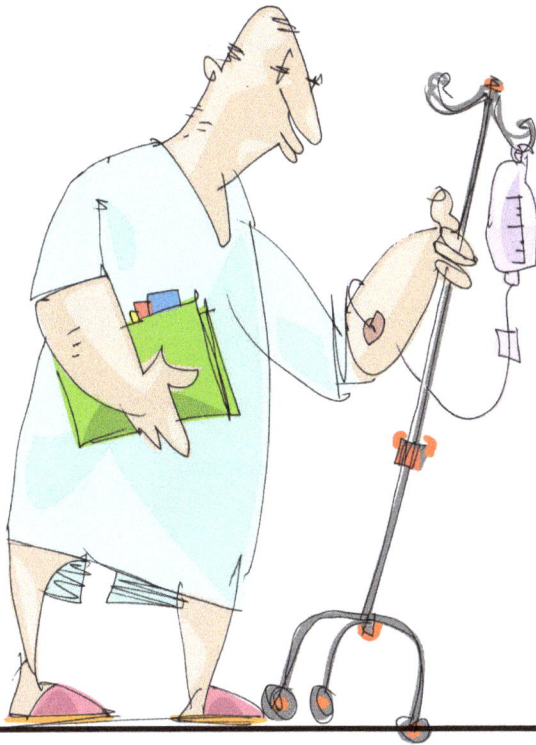

"Warmly affectionate elder abuse."   — Methuselah

"Sadly funny..."   — Sophocles

"The Pet Rock of western literature."   — Anon.

"I don't feel so good."   — John Doe

Top 10 Warnings

1. Hospice is a crock. Keep a jug of water under the bed.
2. Write a will.
4. Hide it.
5. Don't walk toward the light.
6. Did you take your meds today?
7. Are you sure?
8. What happened to Number 3?
9. Eat a pie.
10. If there has ever been something you wanted to do, but didn't for whatever reason, now is the time to do it! Start with this book!

Wisdom of the Aged

PG-65

Dead Is the New Sick
An Insider's Guide to Senility, Paranoia & Curmudgery
Jimmy Huston

www.deadsick.com

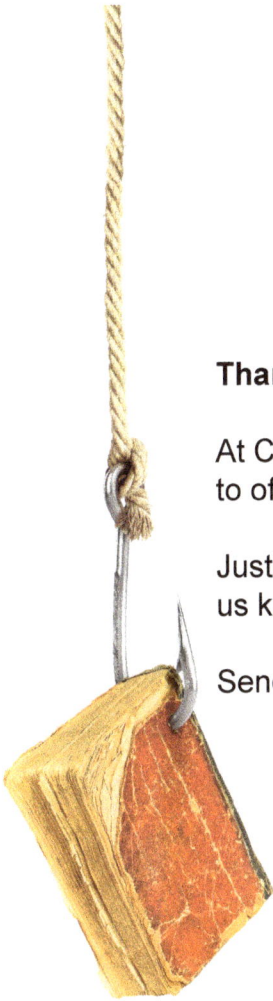

Thanks for buying, borrowing, or swiping this wonderful book.

At Cosworth Publishing we truly appreciate that, and in return, we'd like to offer you one of our E-books absolutely free—and worth every penny.

Just let us know that you want it, and we'll make sure that you get it. Let us know which book you read so we don't send you the same one.

Send an email to *office@cosworthpublishing.com*.

Then, from time to time, we will let you know via email when we have a new book that you might be interested in.

We won't do that very often because we're basically pretty lazy, and we don't produce very many new books.

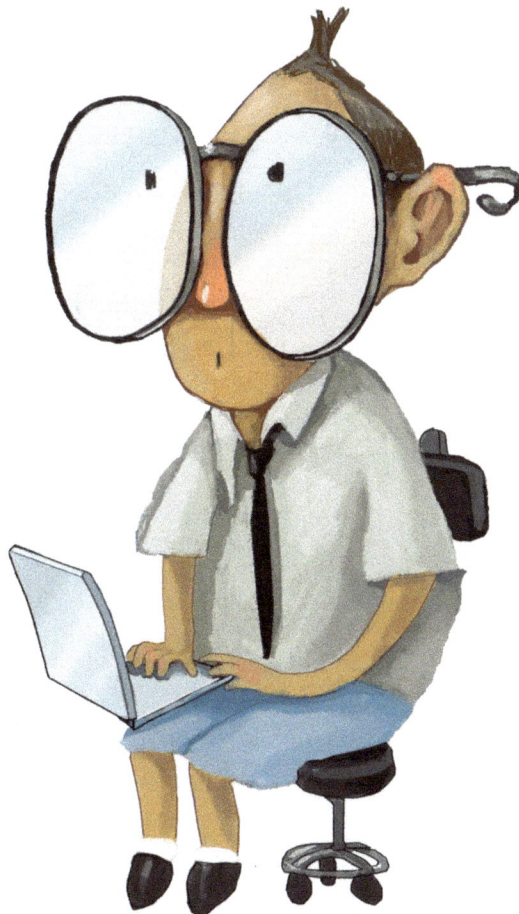

Reviews are usually appreciated.

www.ingramcontent.com/pod-product-compliance
Lightning Source LLC
Chambersburg PA
CBHW042333030426
42335CB00027B/3318